Yoga of Rehab

The Twelve Sutras for Transcending Addiction

Anjali Talcherkar, Ph.D.

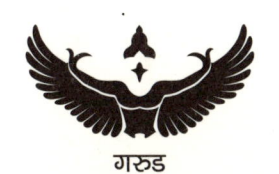

गरुड

Published by
Garuda Prakashan Private Limited
Gurugram, Bharat

www.garudabooks.com

First published in India 2021

Copyright © 2021
Anjali Talcherkar

All rights reserved. No part of this publication may be reproduced or transmitted in any form or by any means, electronic or mechanical, including photocopying, recording, or any information storage or retrieval system, without prior permission in writing from the publishers.

No responsibility for loss caused to any individual or organisation acting on or refraining from action as a result of the material in this publication can be accepted by Garuda Prakashan or the author.

The content of this book is the sole expression and opinion of its author, and not of the publisher. The publisher in no manner is liable for any opinion or views expressed by the author. While best efforts have been made in preparing this book, the publisher makes no representations or warranties of any kind and assumes no liabilities of any kind with respect to the accuracy or completeness of the content and specifically disclaims any implied warranties of merchantability or fitness of use for a particular purpose.

The publisher believes that the content of this book does not violate any existing copyright/intellectual property of others in any manner whatsoever. However, in case any source has not been duly attributed, the publisher may be notified in writing for necessary action.

ISBN: 978-1-942426-54-7

Cover Design: Mahiraj Singh & Kim Feast
Edited by: Diana Drew & Sankrant Sanu
Photography: Samantha Peltz

Printed in India

Dedicated to

His Holiness, Sri Sri Ravi Shankar

Disclaimer

Some names and identifying details have been changed to protect the privacy of individuals. This book is not intended as a substitute for the medical advice of a physician. The reader should consult a physician in matters relating to his/her health and particularly with respect to any symptoms that may require medical attention. Although the author and publisher have made every effort to ensure that the information in this book was correct at press time, the author and publisher do not assume and hereby disclaim any liability to any party for any loss, damage, or disruption caused by errors or omissions, whether such errors or omissions result from negligence, accident, or any other cause.

Contents

Preface   vii

Acknowledgments   xi

Part I: This Book and Me

Introduction   15

My Story   21

Part II: The Twelve Sutras and Me

Sutra One: Surrender   41

Sutra Two: Faith   55

Sutra Three: Willingness   67

Sutra Four: Courage   77

Sutra Five: Trust   87

Sutra Six: Fortitude　　　　　　　　　　97

Sutra Seven: Humility　　　　　　　　　107

Sutra Eight: Forgiveness　　　　　　　　115

Sutra Nine: Responsibility　　　　　　　125

Sutra Ten: Commitment　　　　　　　　133

Sutra Eleven: Liberation　　　　　　　　141

Sutra Twelve: Dharma　　　　　　　　　149

Conclusion　　　　　　　　　　　　　157

Glossary　　　　　　　　　　　　　　158

Notes　　　　　　　　　　　　　　　161

Bibliography　　　　　　　　　　　　166

Preface

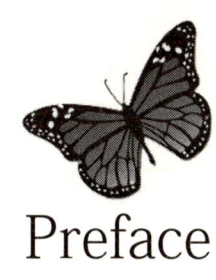

I invite you to plant new thoughts in your mind, to forge a new way of thinking. By recognizing that there is a deeper understanding beyond the surface, you unveil the distorted illusion of the ego-driven mind.

When we cling to the ego's deceptive tricks, we become a pawn of the "egoic puppet master." Living at the level of ego is merely existing. Living from the level of pure consciousness is being. Only by accessing pure consciousness do we find eternal bliss. This book gives you the tools to reach that blissful state, free from addictions.

In times of stress, coping mechanisms, such as abusing addictive substances, become tempting. But such relief is false and futile and it triggers an endless addictive cycle. If we search for answers solely on the surface level, nothing will come of our efforts; transcending addiction requires us to search deeper.

In thoroughly working the twelve sutras, we undergo a complete psychological and spiritual transformation. This change is necessary for us to move beyond the material mind a state of pure consciousness. We can only do this in the present moment. To live fully in the present moment, we must calm the mind, which is churning with unnecessary thoughts. We need to evict those loitering thoughts and supplant them with new thoughts, something that can be achieved through twelve-sutra work and meditation.

These new thoughts may grow into belief. If you act on belief with persistence, it will become habit. These habitual thoughts turn into your character and your awakening to pure consciousness proceeds steadily. This becomes the invitation to progress further.

When thinking expands, being contracts and vice versa. Have you ever observed dancers? They are engrossed in the performance and the rhythm of the music. The activity is occurring in their bodies, not in their minds. People are inspired by the art of dance because dancers are instruments of embodied expression. They are fully in the present moment. The present moment dwells in being. By quieting the mind and cultivating stillness, we gain freedom. Meditation strengthens our inner peace.

Ego identifies with "things" and form; ego spawns superficial dependence on keeping or holding onto worldly things that are constantly changing. Clinging to material objects creates barriers to true happiness. Profound change occurs when we shift from an external orientation to an internal awareness. Stillness within speaks louder than words. Until we explore this stillness, insight lies dormant.

This book is one step on the path to awakening. In the beginning of this process, we hear a still, faint voice, subtle and soft. This voice will transform our outlook, guiding us toward building a tower of love. Before we build this metaphorical tower, however, we need a blueprint. The divine plan is already within us, but we need to enlist the Supreme Architect.

In twelve-step programs, there is a saying that "You cannot transmit something you haven't got." We can give of ourselves once our cup overflows, but how will we replenish our source? By cultivating stillness and practicing meditation, the infinite well of knowledge springs forth from within. Overflowing through prayer and meditation, we find nourishment. Once we fill ourselves with love from the Divine, we are able to give to others. Abundance attracts more abundance. Gratitude keeps us aware of the infinite gifts in this moment. Follow the path with genuine commitment, act with conviction, and remain in the present moment.

Awareness is the most important element in "waking up." Just as, in the physical realm, we use an alarm clock to awaken. Carl Jung once said, "Your vision will become clear only when you look into your heart. Who looks outside, dreams. Who looks inside, awakens."[1]

Following Our Internal Compass

Retreating from chaos and returning to stillness bring us back to our center. There is a compass ingrained in all of us that serves as a guide. People show up at different stages in our lives. These encounters are tools for growth. The Divine places angels as guides on our path. Our job is to follow the guidance and to avoid detours.

When ego drives our life, we crash and blame others. Much of our behavior results from beliefs and ideas based on past experience. If we own our past, we are free to release it and nurture a new reality. Once this process begins, the ego pushes back. We must reach beyond the confines of the ego. Continued deep internal work, via the 12 Sutras, Sudarshan Kriya, yoga, and meditation, promotes a true spiritual awakening. The peace achieved through such work extinguishes the flame of resistance. Through meditation, we tame the ego.

We may never know Truth in a tangible fashion, but it is possible to know a certainty of the Divine Presence. This book is the doorway to knowing that Presence—the Guru Within. I am handing you the key. Will you accept the invitation?

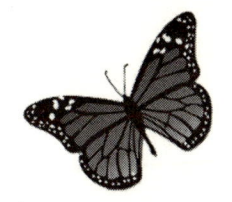

Acknowledgments

First and foremost, utmost gratitude, appreciation, and respects to His Holiness Sri Sri Ravi Shankar. This book was a product of His grace, love, and unwavering guiding light.

Jai Guru Dev.

Heartfelt thanks to all the sponsors, teachers, mentors, guides, friends, and family members who contributed to my journey. Your energy and efforts were invaluable. I want to thank Core Power Yoga, Los Angeles, where I completed my 200-hour yoga teacher training, specifically, the CPY Hollywood studio. Special appreciation to the facilitators and fellow yogis in my cohort!

Much love and gratitude to my editors, Diana Drew and Sankrant Sanu, who brought this book to life creatively, while holding the bigger vision for the book, and all editors who provided their input, suggestions, and expertise. Thank you to Garuda Publishing for taking a chance on a first-time author.

And to those on the path of recovery and beyond....keep going.

Love and Blessings.

Part I

This Book and Me

Introduction

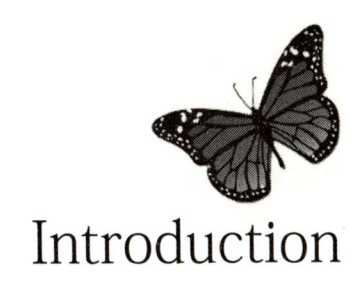

Denial is common among addicted individuals because of the negative stigma associated with the label *addict*. In treatment facilities, clients often cannot move past the stage of denial. Recovery is almost impossible when there is such resistance. People do not want to think of themselves as being bad or their behavior as unacceptable. If we elicit change without labeling or diagnosing, then those struggling with addiction will be more receptive to treatment. Labeling and diagnosing highlight the problem. In *Treating Addiction*, the authors write:

"Neither screening nor diagnosis, however, provides much information about what is actually happening in a particular person's life and substance use, why problems are emerging, and what treatment options would be most appropriate to try. These tasks–to understand the nature and causes of the individual's particular situation and to consider possible routes to change–lie at the heart of evaluation."[1]

I may have been labeled an "addict," but this is not my true nature. This is not who I am, but rather part of how I trained myself to cope with life. This shadow aspect of my personality can be revealed and healed. Embracing this shadow side of myself, instead of being labeled, diagnosed, and forced into a facility to change, has helped me move into acceptance. If we accept that who we really are is not negative, or "bad," then we become open to the healing process and the universe expands to give us exactly what we need to heal. As one person recovers, a community recovers, then society recovers. We need to globally "recover," and this begins with our beliefs about ourselves and who we really are.

Labeling and diagnosing stigmatize us, whereas validation and acceptance empower us. In the long run, labeling becomes highly counterproductive because we are not textbook prototypes and ultimately no one else can tell us what or who we are. Therefore, having a strong sense of Self is necessary for our own evolution. This "knowing" comes from direct experience. When labels are dropped, healing proceeds more smoothly.

Disease and mental illness are human-made concepts that spring from a fear-based system of thought. I did not come into this world with a disease or mental illness. Someone diagnosed me in those terms, then chose to address that "disease" through conventional medicine, rather than helping me find alternative solutions.

Like everyone else, an addicted individual is a very special person who has come into this world with innate gifts and often, extraordinary talents. There should be no negative connotation associated with such a person. The more we seek comfort through drugs—becoming a so-called "hard-core" addict—the more we are actually seeking Higher Consciousness. We are "chasing the guru"–the Divinity within.

Nurturing the Spirit

We sprouted from the seed of Spirit. A seed has all the data in it to know how to bloom: what is green, what is pink, and what fragrance to emit. We came into this world with this seed already planted within us. Our natural intelligence is all we need. Yet this seed gets covered up, almost as if we had sprayed pesticides on our spirit. Throughout life, we acquire stress, negative emotions, and toxins that distort and mutate the seed.

So what is the solution? Raise ourselves organically and purify ourselves. The more we purify ourselves, the more we restore our seed to its natural state. The more we allow our Divine nature to blossom, the sooner we discover our dharma, or life's purpose, and let go of the past.

If you want greater abundance and prosperity in your life, align your thoughts to match your worthiness of that abundance and prosperity. Elevate yourself to live in a higher dimension. When your thoughts are of a higher frequency, your being will tune into that frequency and your physical reality will be transformed. As soon as I truly believed I would be a published author, that conviction reinforced those thoughts and it became my reality. You are fearlessly whole and magnificent; you shine. You just need to know it. Embrace your gifts but know that you possess them to share with others. The Divine has given them to you on layaway. May not be given again (because who really knows that) Discover your truths, your gifts, and share them fearlessly.

The only person who holds onto the past is you. Your ego reminds you of your past to keep you mediocre. One obstacle I faced in early sobriety was the inability to let go of shame and guilt from my past actions. The ego resists transformation because it is an unknown venture. Shed your garments of mediocrity and rock your designer truth! The ego's only purpose is to separate you from your true essence. Don't try to get rid of your ego. Remember, as the guru, Sri Sri Ravi Shankar, states, "Opposite values are complementary."

Duality is often seen as two distinct points of reference, such as fear and love, but they are two sides of the same coin. Without the presence of the ego, we cannot return to the state of love. Simply observe that the ego is there and say, "Next?" OK, you are there—now what? Do not act or react and become paralyzed by the ego. You cannot afford to allow yourself to become separated from your true nature, which is love. Your loving abode is too precious to abandon. It is your responsibility to stay connected to the Divine by focusing on your authenticity. This is the direction in which we are all heading.

We are all moving toward greater integrity and closer connection with the Divine, but how quickly do you want to get there? Haven't you wasted enough energy in endeavors that are only temporarily fulfilling? Are you enjoying the scenery along the way? Do you believe what you see is real? What are your priorities? Seek and ask questions. Are you really satisfied living according to someone else's beliefs? Explore who you really are.

Lessons to Be Learned

So let's look at addiction and relapse. For seven years I kept doing the "relapse and recover" sobriety dance. I would call myself a "chronic relapser." However, after acknowledging the power of thought, I made a decision not to think about myself as a chronic relapser anymore; I made a decision to see myself as whole, perfect, and complete, void of any disease or illness. When I stopped thinking about myself in disease-centered terms, I stopped vocalizing it, and eventually I recovered. I chose to see that there were lessons along the way that I had to learn, and each time my relapse became a little more severe and my "bottom" became lower, the lessons that I derived from those experiences became fundamental to understanding and applying the twelve steps.

Relapse is simply a fall from grace. When we work the twelve sutras, we get closer to grace. When we stop applying spiritual principles to our lives, we "fall from grace." But each time we fall, we are forced to embrace the Twelve Sutras and a spiritual way of life with more fervor.

For addicted individuals, a life devoid of spirituality becomes miserable and unmanageable. So relapse occurs after a sequence of "small slips." When we have hit our "bottom," we are spiritually, mentally, and physically bankrupt. In recovery, first we treat the physical aspect—the body's dependency on the substance. Then we address the entangled mental state, or the so-called "obsessive thinking." Finally, we begin to develop a relationship with Spirit.

In Vedanta—Hindu philosophy—there is something called *prakriti*. This refers to the basic nature of intelligence by which the universe exists and functions. Prakriti is composed of three aspects, or *gunas*. The first guna is *sattva*, or creation. The second guna is *rajas*, or preservation. The third guna is *tamas*, or destruction. *Sattva* is Brahma, the god of creation; *rajas* is Vishnu, the god of preservation; and *tamas* represents Shiva, the god of dissolution or destruction. We all have these three aspects within ourselves and will cycle through these phases at various stages in our life. Many factors contribute to our dominant guna, including diet, the placement of the planets, our surroundings, and people we associate with.

Sattvika individuals are associated with goodness, light, and harmony. They seek answers regarding the origin and truth of material life, and, with proper support, they can reach liberation or *moksha*, which is freedom from worldly existence. They typically consume a vegetarian diet and engage in *sattvic* pleasures, such as yoga and meditation.

Rajasika individuals have a lot of energy and are associated with activity, ambition, and passion. They engage in *rajasic* pleasures, or pleasures of the five senses. These qualities can both support and hinder the soul. In this state, the ego tends to become more distinct because the ego is associated with worldly pursuits.

Tamasika individuals have a lot of inertia, darkness, and insensitivity, and they take the longest to reach liberation. Addicted individuals who don't recover will stay in this state because toxic substances create *tamas*. We come into this world sattvic but through accumulation of internal and external toxins that are not cleansed and released, tamas predominates.

These three gunas are part of a continuous cycle. We revolve through these phases at various points in our life, depending on our priorities, goals, and aspirations. So when we experience sattva, we are spiritually connected, and light radiates from within. We focus on inner life (*navritti*), which is the true source of bliss. When we move into a rajasic phase, our ego takes control again. We look for satisfaction within the world of material things, or form. Many successful, business-minded people stay in the rajasic state, which is often necessary when pursuing material success. The problem arises when attachment to worldly possessions becomes more important than preservation and maintenance of our sattvic nature. When tamas is dominant, we sometimes feel the need to alleviate our inertia, dullness, and darkness with something outside ourselves. We look for sensory pleasure to alleviate the dullness, often through chemical enhancement. Hence, a relapse occurs.

After maturing in recovery, I did not see a relapse as either good or bad. I started to look at it as an opportunity, rather than a crisis. After I got a second DUI and hit a pretty deep bottom, my sponsor told me it was a blessing. I was shocked at her remark! I could not understand how such a catastrophic event could be a blessing; but after witnessing some of the promises coming true in my life thereafter, I understood her logic. When you are in tamas (the destructive phase), the only way to move is toward sattva (the creative phase). This is the nature of the cycle. Shiva destroys but only so that Brahma can create something new. So, do good for yourself and be in sattva.

In Ayurveda, the ancient Hindu system of medicine, these three gunas, which rule the mind, are translated as the *doshas*, or the three energies that circulate through the body and govern physiological activity. The gunas govern the mind and the doshas influence the body; there is an interconnectedness of the mind, body, and spirit. These three doshas are known as *vata, pitta,* and *kapha*. All three doshas must be in balance for overall health and well-being. Addicted individuals need restoration of balance and with this *doshic* balance and harmony, can soar to unimaginable heights in life.

A Note to the Reader

Preceding each of the twelve chapters corresponding to the Twelve Sutras, you'll see a section specifying the Sutra's Principle, Deity, Mantra, Asana, and Meditation. In personally working through the twelve steps from an Eastern/Hindu/Vedantic perspective, I found that each Step/Sutra reflected a key principle and a Hindu Deity. I developed a mantra, and a meditation for each one as well. Finally, based on my training as a certified yoga instructor, I incorporated a yoga pose (asana) that dovetails with each of the Twelve Sutras. These are intended to deepen your understanding of the Twelve Sutra path and make your recovery that much more meaningful.

Namaste

My Story

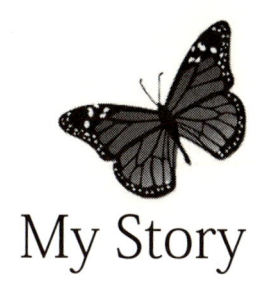

December 24, 2007 found me 60 days sober. I went to a Christmas Eve party with my roommate, having vowed to myself beforehand that I wouldn't have a drink. Not one. Zero. I swore this to myself under my breath as we walked through the door. But as soon as I saw all those people with sloshing liquor glasses, big smiles, and happy gestures, I pulled a drink off a tray and let loose.

Many hours later, loaded on alcohol and relapsed again, I decided to drive to Santa Barbara. Without a second thought, I got in the car and took off. I tried to react, but there was no time. We collided. The next thing I knew, I was carried out of my car on a stretcher and put into an ambulance.

When I woke up in the hospital, I was handcuffed to the bed, and there were two police officers beside me reading me my rights. This wasn't the first occasion I had been read my rights, but I knew this time it was serious. I was in and out of consciousness, but I remember hearing enough to know that they were taking me to jail. I remember being in my cell that night, on the cold metal bunk bed, thinking about how bad things were. I was so caught up in myself that I didn't even stop to think about the people in the car ahead of me that I had hit. They were either injured or dead–I knew that much. But what I couldn't stop feeling—what I couldn't stop aching for— was one more drink, one more line, one more step deeper into that dark hole.

The Early Days

Things were so much simpler when I was a child, when a sense of innocence and amusement permeated my soul. Waking up to a beautiful summer day was incentive enough to live. My days as a child usually began with the tantalizing smell of pancakes and bacon—the staples of a true American breakfast. Surrounded by cornstalks and bean fields, the sights of harvest told me that summer was over and the leaves would soon be changing color. Vibrant greens would turn into magnificent shades of orange and yellow, like a Bob Ross painting. My friend, Jenna and I would explore the woods and head to the creek to catch crawdads or minnows, only to return moments later laughing from my routine fall into the water.

I grew up in a small, rural farm town in Illinois. My brother and I stood out because we were East Indian, and the people in the town were primarily Caucasian. My brother was the intelligent, logical one, destined for medical school. I was the artistic dreamer, in my mind, destined for Hollywood.

My neighborhood friend, Laura, and I would play hopscotch to the soundtrack of *Stand by Me* or set up a lemonade stand, charging a whopping ten cents per cup. The entrepreneurial spirit was alive even in my youngest years. Playing on a tire swing was far more satisfying than surfing the Internet. Gratification came from small things. Our minds weren't constantly distracted by social media or iPhones. We lived in the moment. We were free, with no need to search for fulfillment outside of ourselves. I was content with simplicity and felt a real sense of belonging.

Somewhere along the way, I lost this spirit. It would be years and years before I would find it again.

A Steep Decline

As years passed, my innocence and joy in life seemed to evaporate. I became depressed after my first long-term relationship ended. My parents eventually sent me to a psychiatrist who prescribed antidepressants. Looking back, I realize the medication was just a band-aid to mask the pain; I never dealt with my underlying lack of self-esteem and need for approval and love. At age 15, I entered therapy and would continue seeing many therapists, one after another for years. The talking, the therapy—it just wasn't enough. I needed something more, something to numb my pain— an instant fix. I turned to alcohol and drugs.

I gravitated to the older crowd in school. They were "cool," and I desperately wanted to be liked by them. All the older kids partied, and it just seemed like the logical thing to do. I began hanging out with them on the weekends, going to keg parties in the country with no city lights, no paved roads, just open cornfields. We would speed through the country night, drinking Keystone Light, and singing along to songs on the radio. We called it, "road-tripping." We'd explore the countryside—nothing but endless country miles that we would map out and drive through all night long.

The town we lived in had a central square with a bar on every corner, and often we would meet each other there throughout the night to find out whose parents were away so we could throw a party. When we ran out of alcohol, we would have to persuade people over twenty one to buy us more. We would park next to the local gas station and just wait. As long as we bought our suppliers something or gave them a little extra cash, it was never a problem. My negotiation skills developed at a young age.

Those nights ended in blackouts and excruciating morning-after hangovers. At one point, I was so intoxicated that I could not stop vomiting and had to be taken to the hospital. I lied to my parents and told them I had food poisoning. These were early signs of alcoholism, but I didn't know it then, and I would continue to torture myself for the next 20 years.

Alcohol has been described as a gateway drug, and for me this was certainly true. Soon, I was introduced to marijuana. I had a "posse" in high school—Me, A, and C. We liked to call ourselves the "Buddha Lovin' Trio." We wore flannel shirts, rocked Doc Martins, and listened to the Grateful Dead. Our whole identity revolved around drugs. Eventually, hallucinogens came into the picture, and I started experimenting with acid and mushrooms. And then came the designer "club" drugs—ecstasy and cocaine. Bumps and lines became my first language. The drugs, the guys, the thrill of the rush—it was all fun and games until it just wasn't anymore.

I was on the fast track to disaster, but I just saw it as being young and having fun. The truth is, some people may be able to experiment with drugs and then grow out of it. I didn't know at the time that I had an addictive personality; I was different from others, an extremist who couldn't help pushing the limits. I had become a totally different person than the young, innocent girl. The alcohol and drug use only exacerbated my depression. I needed the drugs to feel good, but when they wore off, I was miserable.

In Denial

Before my senior year of high school, my parents sent me to an outpatient adolescent treatment program. I stayed there for the summer and lived with a psychiatrist who was a friend of the family. I was only 16 and had no clue about recovery. More importantly, I didn't think I had a problem. To me, my drug use was just experimental, and I wasn't an addict. At that program, I was first introduced to Alcoholics Anonymous. We sat in a circle, facing one another. Our parents were there. We had to state our name and our disease. I hesitated. I said, "My name is Anjali and…I am an alcoholic." I looked over at my mom and tears fell from her eyes. I felt ashamed and refused to believe this was true. I was in serious denial. The stigmatizing began early for me, something from which my recovery journey has brought freedom.

Because I did not believe I had a problem, I could not accept the help that was offered to me. After the program ended, I happily returned to my old stomping grounds and fell back into my established routine. One of the things we had learned at the outpatient program was that we needed to change our friends and find sober people with whom to hang out. I wasn't willing to drop my old buddies, and history just seemed to repeat itself. I began to get deeper into the drug scene and school didn't matter. Alcohol and drugs had become my priority; everything else stood in the way.

I had an endless supply of my parents' cash; a drug habit like mine wasn't cheap - why would I want to stop? I thought I could make a little money by selling marijuana out of my dorm room. But I usually smoked up all my profits. I had no real friends, only acquaintances who were part of my party scene. All my life I was running from myself, full of fear. I was afraid that I would fail or that I wouldn't live up to my potential, that I wouldn't make my parents proud or fulfill my purpose in life.

Chasing the Guru

On a visit home to see my parents, I was complaining of neck pain due to excessive exercise. My dad took me to his office and gave me some pain medication. He opened up the cupboard and gave me some sample packets of Tramadol, a pill that produced the same effects as an opiate. I fell in love. A simple pill that could make me instantly euphoric—this was the feeling I had been searching for my whole life. Some people refer to opiate addiction as "chasing the dragon." I was chasing the guru. The drug became my replacement for Divinity. I was looking to fulfill that part of me that felt empty on the inside. The pill emulated the feeling of the Divine. At that point, I had found what would eventually become the center of my universe. All I had to do was pop a pill and wait—anything to change how I was feeling.

There were no consequences in my life yet, other than emotional instability, so I had no reason to stop my destructive behavior. I went through cycles of feeling good, then feeling completely depressed. The partying continued, but I knew I needed to do more with my life. I got a job as a manager at a brokerage firm. I was placing buy/sell orders of Disney shares by day and doing drugs by night.

I was getting deeper into pills. I started buying Vicodin wherever I could find it—five or six here and there. One of my coworkers would give me some of her Xanax if I would cover her shifts. My habit started out with one or two Vicodin a day and a Xanax at night to sleep. I was digging myself deeper into a dark hole of despair. One night, I took several Vicodin, and got scared that I had taken too much. My friend rushed me to the hospital, and I ended up in the psychiatric ward for the first time. I felt a sense of comfort, like I was safe. I saw a psychiatrist and she released me the next day.

My parents felt I should start seeing a psychiatrist on a regular basis and get on antidepressants. Once again, the answer was to medicate the problem. More pills, more pills, more pills! The drug habit was starting to wreak havoc on my personal life as well, but it wasn't enough to stop. I started experimenting with stronger pills and got into Oxycontin. I would chop them up and snort the powder. It enhanced my creativity and I would paint for hours. I also met a guy who had just been released from jail and he re-introduced me to cocaine. I began spending all my money on drugs. The cocaine kept me up and the Oxycontin brought me down. It was an ideal combination. I picked up a cigarette smoking habit, which only added to my destructive addictive tendencies.

One night I drank a lot of alcohol and took some pills. I got violently ill and passed out on my floor. Right at that moment, my friend called me and I could barely answer the phone. Sensing that something was wrong, she rushed over to my apartment and took me to the ER. I was sick the whole way to the hospital. I survived my first overdose thanks to her; she was an angel in disguise. I was released from the hospital after getting some fluids, and the next day I bought some more OxyContin. The insanity continued.

I started seeing a new psychiatrist and also started seeing a therapist who suggested I go to a 30-day treatment program. I almost laughed at that idea. I didn't have that severe of a problem. In my eyes, my life was still manageable. To me, I had just lost my sense of direction in life.

Then, I started buying pills on the Internet, including Hydrocodone and Ativan. I managed to find my roommate's codeine in the medicine cabinet. Anything I could get my hands on was fair game. I became depressed again and would lie in bed, comatose from the pills. My antidepressants didn't seem to be working anymore. I called my psychiatrist and he suggested I go to detox. My life was starting to become unmanageable.

A Glimmer of Hope

I was severely underweight and depressed, so my mom thought it would be good for me to get away for a while; she took me to India. Surely, leaving the country would keep me sober. We decided to stay at my mom's guru's ashram, a place of solitude and worship. His name was Sri Sri Ravi Shankar, not to be confused with the singer. He was the founder of the Art of Living Foundation. I had a dream about him a couple of years before actually meeting him. In the dream, he squeezed my hand tightly, and he asked me what I wanted. I didn't know what to say, and he kept squeezing my hand tighter and tighter until I said, "knowledge and wisdom." He finally let go of my hand, and then I woke up.

Sri Sri told my mother to bring me to the ashram for an Ayurvedic panchakarma treatment. It was rare to get any personal time with him. The ashram was beautiful and serene. It was full of greenery, which reminded me of the vibrant colors and ease of my youth. In the morning, I would hear people chanting and praying. Some would be in solitude, meditating. There were monkeys swinging from trees and peacocks in the garden. There were no televisions, radios, or laptops. This was a completely different way of life. It was a matter of learning to just be, free from distractions. It was a place where you could connect to the Divine Presence.

Initially, I was going stir crazy; I did not know how to be with myself. I couldn't talk on the phone, and there was no entertainment. I had to find joy in the small things. I would walk around and ask some of the workers what to do. They would tell me to go feed the peacocks or cut vegetables. I thought that was silly. What I now see is that they were trying to teach me to be of service, to look beyond my own needs and attend to the needs of others.

I went to the medical clinic where I was seen by an Ayurvedic doctor. He read my pulse and told me I had incurred extreme damage to my central nervous system, most likely from the drugs. He also told me that I had chronic digestive problems, and my stomach had actually been hardened from the pills. Every day I received oil treatments and a massage and was put on a very strict vegetarian diet consisting of lentils and soft, easily digestible foods. The ashram was sprawling, so I got plenty of exercise walking from one end to the other. At night, we all assembled in the new hall to sing. Then the Guru would share some knowledge for the evening. People were awestruck by his presence, how he seemed to float when he walked. It was mystifying. And when I was close to him, it was hard to even speak. Many people would simply start crying. He had a demeanor that made me feel like I was completely taken care of, that I need not have any worries. We would all wait outside his little hut just for the chance to see him. One day I was standing in the front as he was walking up. He saw me, and a wide smile came upon his face. He gave me a huge hug. It was as though I was reuniting with a very dear friend.

One night my mother and I heard a knock on the door. It was 1:00 in the morning. The messenger told us that the Guru was requesting we meet with him. There were thousands of people staying in the ashram. How had he known what room we were in? We walked to his little hut and sat in front of him. He knew I was struggling with addiction. He looked at me and said, "Just get up and go to yoga in the morning. Brush your teeth and go. You like yoga." I could not make the connection at the time but years later my destiny to become a yoga teacher was realized. A guru always knows your path.

I decided to take an introductory course where I learned a breathing technique called *Sudarshan Kriya Yoga* (SKY). It seemed that it might help in my battle with depression and addiction. After taking the course, I noticed an improvement in my overall mood; I felt happy and less fearful. Our trip to India ended, and we reluctantly headed back to the States. I was hoping this would be the spiritual awakening I needed to finally get sober. Without following a program of recovery, I managed to find some pills in my house, and, without thinking twice, I popped a couple in my mouth.

I started doing the Sudarshan Kriya (SKY) once again and managed to quit smoking for a while. It was interesting to observe that consistent practice of SKY played a big role in the release of addictions in my life. At this point, I was living in Minnesota attending the Aveda Institute. I asked the founder of Aveda, an avid meditator, how to manifest my dreams. He told me to meditate twice a day. Taking his advice, I began a meditation practice. I would meditate on things I wanted to accomplish in life, trying to make my dreams a reality. For instance, I had been thinking about moving to Hollywood for quite some time to pursue my makeup career. I wanted to be a celebrity makeup artist and work on movie sets.

I accepted work doing makeup and hair on a Bollywood movie in Detroit for the summer. On the movie set I made a contact who had a connection in Hollywood. The contact was shooting an independent film and looking for interns. I showed an interest and got an offer to work on the film. Within a month, I had booked my flight and packed up all my belongings to move, feeling that the meditation had helped manifest my dream. Meditation is the medium to manifestation.

A Dangerous Combination

Shortly after I relocated to California, my parents divorced and my mom followed me to California. One morning, I bought a bottle of Sky vodka at 9:00 a.m. when the liquor store opened and snorted the remaining specs of white powder I had purchased the night before. For an active addict, coke and alcohol always complement each other nicely. As soon as I felt too amped from the powder, I would counter the effects with the alcohol. It was a vicious cycle of highs and lows, followed by feelings of hopelessness and despair, leaving me wanting to end my life. The only way out of it was to repeat the cycle. An active drug addict's life is like a bad rerun.

The next thing I knew, I was in the hospital. When they finally took the muzzle off, I saw that the policewoman was in the room with me. Miraculously, I managed to stay out of jail that night. But my destructive behavior was getting out of control and impending doom was near. The ugly cycle of addiction continued, because I had to use more drugs to forget how I was harming myself, and to purge the accumulated feelings of guilt and shame.

My First AA Meeting

A therapist in LA suggested I go to AA. I went to my first AA meeting at Radford Hall, *Big Book of Alcoholics Anonymous* in hand. The speakers inspired me. They each talked about the promises coming true in their life. They no longer felt self-pity or that yearning for external fulfillment because they had found spiritual relief, enabling them to pursue and realize their dreams.

My therapist introduced me to Carl Jung and Jungian psychology. I had become fascinated with the field of psychology because of my own therapy through the years. I was interested in the workings of the mind, and I had a deep need to understand myself. I was continually searching for who I was because I didn't really know myself. I had no identity outside of drugs.

I had a very good connection with this therapist. She had been sober for several years, and I admired that. She encouraged me to keep attending meetings and to stay sober. For the next five years I went in and out of AA. I would get 30 or 60 days sober and then relapse. I never took the program seriously because I had yet to face any severe consequences. From the outside, my life seemed to be in order. I had occasional run-ins with the police, and had been to the mental hospital, and had a DUI conviction, but I didn't attribute this to my drinking or using.

Instead I saw these episodes as stemming from severe depression or bipolar syndrome, a couple of the diagnoses I had been given by psychiatrists over the years. However, now as a clinician working with addicted individuals, I see that it's difficult to obtain an accurate diagnosis when someone is actively using drugs; the symptoms mimic mental disorders.

I decided to go back to school to get my master's degree in psychology at Antioch University of Los Angeles; I applied for the fall quarter and got accepted. I was 60 days clean and sober and confident that I had it together this time. I started school and loved what I was learning. I became fascinated by Jung and began reading books on the unconscious and the shadow self. I recognized in some way that I was trying to uncover my own shadow. I put all my energy into school and neglected my recovery program.

But AA wasn't enough for my case. I eventually started buying extra-strength Vicodin from a guy I had met on a film set while doing extra work. I would go to my chemical dependency class high on pills! The rest of the time, I was also high on pills. I couldn't write papers without popping pills; I couldn't function without them. They were the first thing I thought of when I woke up and the last thing I did before I went to bed. Pills controlled my life. I was confident and outgoing, but this was all an illusion. Deep down, I was afraid that people would find out what was really going on and learn that I was trying to escape reality.

My life had become truly unmanageable, and that was obvious to everyone else. I had been in and out of court for a year, awaiting sentencing for my second DUI. I was eventually convicted of a DUI felony, but had a good lawyer, so instead of jail time, I managed to get four months of house arrest. That one intoxicated night driving to Santa Barbara haunted me and the consequences were now a harsh reality.

Still oblivious to the consequences of my actions, I violated my curfew and had to return to court to renegotiate my sentence. Standing in the courtroom in an orange jumpsuit with both ankles shackled, I finally had a moment of clarity that I had truly hit rock bottom. I glanced at my mother, who had tears running down her cheeks. This certainly could not be the same daughter who was once a bubbling ball of energy and laughter. Finally, the judge decided that I needed to do the actual jail time to learn my lesson.

In Jail

When I arrived at the Santa Barbara County Jail, I experienced a sinking feeling in my gut. I had no idea how I would survive or how I would maintain my sanity locked up for four months. Being treated like a caged animal would make anyone go mad. But I had no choice; I could not talk my way out of this, nor would my parents bail me out.

You never truly appreciate freedom until it is taken away. The women in my cell seemed rough around the edges. We slept on triple-decker, iron bunk beds with paper-thin mattresses. They kept the pods extremely cold and only gave us a thin sheet to cover up with at night.

There is nothing more degrading than having to take communal showers with 15 other women. Some of them scanned me like they were eyeing their next victim. Our daily regimen was 4:00 a.m. wake up, chores, checks, and the occasional game of spades to pass the time. My anxiety would finally dissipate around 9:00 p.m., knowing I had survived another day of verbal abuse from the correctional officers. At night, I would be awakened to the sound of women screaming from their nightmares. Finally, I received word that my lawyer had arranged a deal with the judge, and I was released from jail. After this incident, I realized I really needed to get sober.

Another Try at Recovery & Tragedy

A few months later, I entered detox before entering yet another rehabilitation program. I enjoyed the detox drugs just as much as the good ones from my addiction. A month following detox, I went to a rehab facility in Santa Barbara called Casa Serena, which means "serene house." Upon arrival, I was greeted by a group of girls who were quite friendly and welcoming. Initially, it was overwhelming. There were rules and chores, and I certainly was not used to abiding by any of them. We woke up at 6:30 a.m. and had a strict regimen to follow all day. The day included morning walks and meditation, recovery groups, meals, and AA meetings.

This was where my true journey to recovery began. The executive director had an admirable spiritual essence about her that attracted me. She gave me a book on Buddhism and the 12-steps, which helped deepen my spiritual awareness. I did well at this facility and was making progress, able to stay clean and sober. I began doing yoga and meditating daily. Routine is very good for addressing addiction because consistency is lacking. Two weeks before I was to graduate from the program, I decided to leave and head to Los Angeles. I entered Magnolia Place, a sober-living colony—a less structured environment than an actual treatment facility. We were required to go to 12 AA meetings a week if we were not working.

While in Magnolia Place, I met a guy in AA who was also in recovery from addiction. We began to hang out more and more and were going to meetings together. We became exclusive and despite suggestions from others in recovery not to get into a relationship in my first year of sobriety, I did. Eventually, we lost track of our individual priorities, especially recovery. In October 2009, we decided to go to Las Vegas and get married on a whim. We hopped in the car and stopped at a gas station to celebrate on the way. We purchased a bottle of vodka and relapsed on the drive to Vegas.

After we got married and returned to Los Angeles, I went to Chicago to spend the holidays with my father. In February 2010, I attended an AA meeting, having not heard from my husband for three days. I had a suspicion that he was struggling, but he didn't usually just disappear. When I got back to my father's home, he asked me to sit down. My father told me that my husband had died from a heroin overdose. A needle was in his arm when he was found.

I was emotional and did not know how to react. I was not able to grasp the reality of the situation. I disassociated from experiencing the overwhelming feelings of grief. Even though I hadn't known him very long, it was a heartbreaking situation to see anyone go like that. But this is the reality of addiction. I just didn't think I would experience it so up close and personal.

The Journey to Recovery

After my husband's death, I was struggling to stay sober, so I entered Friendly House, the oldest women's recovery home in the United States. I selected a sponsor and began working the 12-steps again. Slowly, things started to improve, which is what usually happens when you actually work the steps and apply them to your daily life. My sponsor personally knew Marianne Williamson, a spiritual luminary, author, and lecturer, and she asked me if I wanted to intern for her. I had recently read Ms. Williamson's first book, *A Return to Love*, and proceeded to read the rest of her books. I felt a strong connection to her words, and her work catapulted me onto my own spiritual quest. It was amazing to be in the presence of such an inspiring and enlightened woman. I learned much from that experience; I also became involved in the Art of Living Foundation and started practicing the Sudarshan Kriya (SKY) breathing meditation again. I found solace in yoga, silent meditation courses, and my meditation practice. Something on the inside was blossoming. I began to get in touch with the Divine within. The combination of working the 12 steps, the SKY practice, and meditation was a magic antidote.

The Art of Living Foundation and its sister organization, International Association for Human Values (IAHV) teaches breathing and meditation techniques that improve overall physical and mental health. I was drawn to the practices and the Vedic philosophies that undergirded them, especially that of Ayurveda. I had seen how Ayurveda had helped me somewhat with my addiction while I stayed at the ashram in India. I began to study Ayurveda again, and learned that an imbalance in the doshas contributes to addiction, and for that matter, all diseases.

By consistently doing my spiritual practices, following an Ayurvedic regimen of adopting a specific diet according to my dosha type, doing the Sudarshan Kriya, and applying the 12-steps, I was able to wean myself off all the medication I had been prescribed. I had been seeing psychiatrists for 20 years and was never able to be completely medication-free. Many people were skeptical about my decision to discontinue my medication, but I knew in my heart that I had to free myself from any dependency to mind-altering chemicals. Through my own 12-step work, I also found that I could not have conscious contact with the Divine if I was still seeking a crutch to alleviate my problems. I began incorporating the AOL principles into my 12-step work which resulted in a manuscript, or guidebook, to help people free themselves from addiction.

Nothing truly magnificent in life ever develops without some risk. My inner voice was telling me to trust and rely completely on my Guru. There was a pull to return to the joy of my childhood, before addiction stole my innocence and interrupted my purpose. Thus, my inquiry into Eastern science and holistic medicine grew. I also became fascinated with Vedanta, the Hindu philosophy of life.

Through a consistent regimen of Ayurveda, Art of Living courses, and the Twelve Sutras, I was able to recover. This journey has allowed me to have a truly fulfilling connection to the Divine Source, and this remains the center of abundance in my life. All external abundance emerges from this well. All forms of genius and creativity spring from this space. Eventually, I experienced a profound spiritual awakening, which facilitated a full break from addiction. My path to enlightenment brought me to my doctoral journey, and a desire to study my recovery by completing a PhD in Integrative Medicine. As I progressed in my own recovery, continued growth led to a release of all labels and previous "addict" identity, ultimately, transcending addiction.

Part II

The Twelve Sutras and Me

SUTRA ONE

PRINCIPLE: Surrender

DEITY: Padmavati

MANTRA: *Om Svaha*
(I surrender my mind, intelligence, and ego to the Lord)

ASANA: *Balasana* (child's pose)

MEDITATION: (Repeat this to yourself throughout the day).

"All of me, I surrender to Thee."

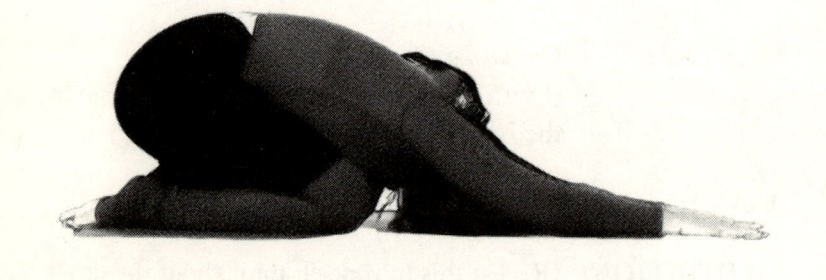

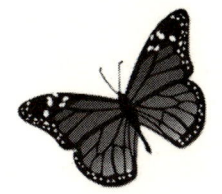

Sutra One: Surrender

*I admit I am more powerful than
the addiction, and that my life is manageable*

You can struggle or you can surrender. You can fight or you can admit defeat. You have tried time and time again, but you always seem to fall short. Somehow, your well-thought-out plans never come to fruition. This is because Universal Consciousness, or universal law, trumps human-made laws and beliefs. You can continue to struggle and try to manage and maintain control, but you will find these attempts futile in the long run.

The universe shines on you when your will is in sync with the good of humanity or aligned with the collective. The universe works in favor of those who believe in promoting the common good. For example, once I truly began to home in on my life's purpose and serve those suffering from addiction, obstacles in my path began to fall away. I had a felony conviction on my record and prospective employers did extensive background checks. Even though I was somewhat unemployable because of this violation, the universe placed me exactly where I needed to be: working in a nondisease-model, holistic treatment center.

Surrendering is much more cost-and-time-effective as a way to make our dreams a reality. Recall the fable of the lion and the lamb. The lion represents our courage, but the passivity of the lamb also exemplifies strength. It took both courage and strength for you to get to this point; now relax, let go.

The practice of yoga is a beautiful example of this dance. It takes muscular strength and mental determination to hold certain postures, but it also requires the ability to relax and allow the tension to dissipate. No asana practice would be complete without the final and most important posture, *sivasana*, where we integrate the activity of the practice, letting go and allowing the body to come to a state of full relaxation.

Finding Strength in Surrender

Opposite values are complementary, meaning that you cannot attempt surrender without a vast reserve of courage. Surrendering takes strength and once you are able to bow down, relinquishing control, the possibility of transformation emerges. You need this shift in awareness to create a new life. Surrendering is the beginning of living life to its fullest.

I was once in the emergency room with a client who had suffered a terrible trauma and recently lost her daughter. She was numbing herself with opiates because of the excruciating physical and emotional pain. She looked at me and said, "I'm just looking for a reason to wake up in the morning." Obviously, this woman could continue to struggle and sedate herself, or she could simply surrender. She was trying to control the pain in an attempt to control the suffering, but that strategy was not working. I looked at her and replied, "Just surrender." She raised her head and whispered, "Surrender to what?"

It does not matter what you surrender to, but by loosening the grip of control, you allow a force beyond your rational mind to help you. When the end seems near, it is only the beginning if we hand the reins over to a Power that can steer us in a positive direction. We sometimes think we are losing by surrendering. As a wise woman once told me, "surrendering is coming over to the winning side."

There is strength and wisdom in this nonaction. In the beginning of a yoga practice, we start in *balasana*, or child's pose.

Our body is on the floor in a fetal position with the forehead resting on the ground. An infant needs the guidance of its mother in the early stages of life. Similarly, in recovery, we need to surrender and allow a Power that knows best to guide us.

Exerting control limits possibility. At one point in my life, I was fixated on creating a relationship with someone whom I felt was the "one." I was doing everything in my power to make it work, but it just wasn't happening because I was trying to force it. In hindsight, I can see that the universe had much bigger plans for me. I was limiting the possibility of having a beautiful experience of love and union by thinking that I could only achieve it with this particular person.

When we truly want something, the universe will respond with one of three answers: "Yes," "Not right now," or "I have something better in mind for you." The greater the possibility, the better life can be. There are numerous ways in which love can flow into our lives. Beautiful music is made by a wide array of instruments. Similarly, partnerships are simply different instruments harmonizing to create a love song.

Life alone is unmanageable because it is filled with uncertainty. How can we manage uncertainty? We see people doing it every day; thus the inevitable question: Why can't we? One artist said it perfectly: "You can plan a pretty picnic, but you can't predict the weather." A Yiddish proverb echoes that sentiment: "Man plans and God laughs."

I get uncomfortable when people ask me what my plans are because most of the time, my plans change. I set intentions, move with determination, and surrender to the results. The Bhagavad Gita states:

"You have the right to work, but for the work's sake only. You have no right to the fruits of work. Desire for the fruits of work must never be your motive in working. Never give way to laziness, either. Perform every action with you heart fixed on the Supreme Lord. Renounce attachment to the fruits. Be even-tempered in success and failure: for it is this evenness of temper which is meant by yoga.

Work done with anxiety about results is far inferior to work done without such anxiety, in the calm of self-surrender. Seek refuge in the knowledge of Brahma. They who work selfishly for results are miserable."[1]

Spontaneity tends to guide my life. As a student of yoga, I have learned the valuable tool of nonattachment, *vairagya*. I used to be very attached to my environment and surroundings, but the Divine will challenge you when you get caught in this mind-set. As soon as I became comfortable, I would be offered another job in a completely different area or a better opportunity would present itself, requiring me to shift my surroundings. One thing that is always certain is change. When you learn to ride this current, life becomes much more fluid and things happen naturally. So, when someone asks, "Where do you see yourself a year from now?" My answer is "happy." I see myself as happy, and wherever, whenever, with whomever that works out is fine, as long as it is aligned with the universe's plan.

In Sutra One, once we accept that our true Self is more powerful than our addiction, we surrender, and are free to begin living instead of just existing. Out of that very acceptance comes liberation of the soul.

Discovering Our Destiny

We spend a lot of time running from ourselves because we don't want to be who we think we are. But if we stop running and find the courage to face ourselves honestly, we discover that our true essence is nothing to run from; rather, it is something to embrace. When we discover who we really are, life becomes full, rich, pleasant, and vibrant. This is the catalyst for uncovering and discarding whatever no longer serves our greatest good. The very fact that we are here in human form means that we have a unique mission or destiny to fulfill.

Working the Twelve Sutras leads us in the direction of discovering our *dharma*, or life's purpose, and once we begin to recognize ourselves and our dharma, life blossoms. We no longer shudder with fear, closed inside the bud. We open up to what the world has to offer. We awaken to our Higher Self. We become solid and grounded.

The ebb and flow of the external world we live in no longer sway us. We are able to look beyond duality and accept that everything is occurring in a natural divine order. We no longer run from craving to aversion, or the "I want/I don't want" state of mind. Active addiction is nothing more than this vicious mental cycle being played out—enhancing pleasure and minimizing pain. It is human nature to want to feel good and avoid discomfort. We seek the dopamine rush that drugs provide at any cost and forsake daily responsibilities, such as jobs. The immediate pleasure overrules the responsibility, which carries a long-term return but also requires effort, discipline, and commitment. In the ancient Hindu texts, there are two concepts: *shreyas* vs *preyas*. According to a verse in Kathopanishad (1.2.2), "From between *shreyas* (that which is good to the Higher Self) and *preyas* (that which is pleasing to the senses) the wise one always chooses the *shreyas*."[2] We can't expect fruit if we don't tend to the tree, and the phenomenon of addiction is similar to stripping an orchard of all its fruit.

This acceptance and surrender cannot happen if we feel that we must be in control. We are not the doers. So the unmanageability comes from wanting to remain the same because we fear change. But change is inevitable, and the world of materiality is *anitya* (impermanence). Suffering comes from being tied to this illusion. In fact, the cycle of birth and death relates to this attachment to *maya*, or illusion. Nothing we experience through our five senses will remain constant. In active addiction, the senses literally become overwhelmed by sense objects.

One addiction that I had a particularly hard time overcoming was the addiction to sugar. Cookies and ice cream teased my taste buds to the point that the immediate gratification of the pleasurable taste outweighed the consequences of the inevitable crash I would experience moments after I consumed the substance. My sense of taste became enraptured by the object of my desire—sugar. But the feeling of immediate gratification would never have lasted and even if I experienced this temporary pleasure over and over, it would have never been enough. Those in the rooms of AA often mention the phrase, "One is too many and a thousand is never enough."

Dis-ease and Ego

My search to understand the mind began when I started questioning the dis-ease of addiction and how I could function with this "ism"—alcoholism. The deeper question I asked myself was this: "Who or what is the 'I' that has this 'ism'?" When I was introduced to *A Course in Miracles* after interning for internationally acclaimed author and spiritual luminary Marianne Williamson, the idea of having a "dis-ease" seemed to be a rather gloomy, fearful outlook. So if addiction is a dis-ease, what aspect of our existence is not at ease? The ego.

Ego is the sum of our conditioning. It is the part of us that doesn't want to be a team player. It has a need to stand out, show off, and dance to its own beat. The ego will often succumb to temptation because it is bound to the material, physical plane. It loves worldly success. It craves respect and admiration. I would assume that my ego is powerless. What true power could such a primitive, superficial identity hold?

Beyond Ego

However, when we move deeper into our true nature, the *atman*, beyond ego and mind, we discover that our power has no limitations. When we learn to align our thoughts and actions from our core, we gain the power we need to carry out miracles. Padmavati is believed to be a form of Lakshmi, the Goddess of wealth and abundance. In Hindu darshan or vision, Lakshmi was Devi, the mother and source of the universe.

Surrendering to the Source, as a child relents to its mother, is a powerfully passive act. In the mother's arms, a child feels completely secure and cared for. Lakshmi represents detachment from the material world; transcendence from the outer reality. Similarly, in the act of surrendering to Divinity, we rise above and find eternal peace. In Hindu mysticism, the goddess Padmavati represents "she who emerged from the lotus." The lotus is considered a sacred flower—it grows in the swamp but is above and untouched by it. Its unfolding petals represent expansion of the soul. When we go beyond ego and mind, our *atman*, or soul, is revealed.

The disease model has produced a huge following among adherents of Alcoholics Anonymous and Narcotics Anonymous. Although Bill Wilson, AA's founder, never stated that alcoholism was a disease, he laid the groundwork for a form of recovery that many have embraced. The American Psychiatric Association declared alcoholism a disease in 1965; the American Medical Association followed suit in 1966.

Alcoholics Anonymous and Spirituality

The founders of *Alcoholics Anonymous*, Bill Wilson and Dr. Bob Smith, were both alcoholics in 1930s America, unable to achieve sustained abstinence despite their Christian faith and membership in the Oxford Group.

"The Oxford Group was a religious movement popular in the United States and Europe in the early 20th century. Members of the Oxford Group practiced a formula of self-improvement by performing self-inventory, admitting wrongs, making amends, using prayer and meditation, and carrying the message to others."[3]

In the 1930s an American, seeking help for his alcohol addiction, paid a visit to Carl Jung. At the time Jung thought the visitor's condition was hopeless and suggested the man could find relief "through a vital spiritual experience." Jung directed him to the Oxford Group. The American, Roland H., joined the group and brought with him Edwin T. Both men used the principles espoused by the Oxford Group and found recovery. Eventually an old friend of Edwin's named Bill W. asked for help to overcome his own addiction using the same principles. Bill was resistant to the Oxford's principles and ended up in a New York City hospital. It was while he was hospitalized that Bill had his transcendent awakening.

For Bill this transcendent experience released him from the depths of dispair and "he was left knowing that life was meaningful, not hopeless, senseless, and chaotic." In reflection, Wilson wrote, "A great peace stole over me and I thought, 'No matter how wrong things seem to be, they are all right. Things are all right with God and His world.'"[4] Wilson began an educational journey looking into the transcedental experience that led him to the work of William James. He later received a letter from Jung many years after his white light experience. The letter referred to the patient (Roland H.) that he had been unable to help who he later recommended to the Oxford Group:

"What I really thought about was the result of many experiences with men of this kind. His craving for alcohol was the equivalent on a low level, of the spiritual thirst of our being for wholeness, expressed in medieval language: the union with God. The only right and legitimate way to such an experience is that it happens to you in reality, and it can only happen to you when you walk on a path, which leads you to higher understanding. You might be led to that goal by an *act* of grace or through a personal and honest contact with friends, or through a higher education of the mind beyond the confines of mere rationalism."[5]

Alcoholics Anonymous was born with the basic principles of "honesty, love, purity, and unselfishness" that Bill borrowed from the Oxford Group. Eventually Wilson arrived at his twelve-step program, which includes the following:

1) We admitted we were powerless over alcohol, that our lives had become unmanageable.
2) Came to believe that a Power greater than ourselves could restore us to sanity.
3) Made a decision to turn our will and our lives over to the care of God *as we understood Him.*
4) Made a searching and fearless moral inventory of ourselves.
5) Admitted to God, to ourselves, and to another human being the exact nature of our wrongs.

6) Were entirely ready to have God remove all these defects of character.
7) Humbly asked Him to remove our shortcomings.
8) Made a list of all persons we had harmed and became willing to make amends to them all.
9) Made direct amends to such people wherever possible, except when to do so would injure them or others.
10) Continued to take personal inventory and when we were wrong promptly admitted it.
11) Sought through prayer and meditation to improve our conscious contact with God, *as we understood Him,* praying only for knowledge of His will for us and the power to carry that out.
12) Having had a spiritual awakening as the result of these steps, we tried to carry this message to alcoholics, and to practice these principles in all our affairs.

In Vedanta, the orthodox system of Hindu philosophy that translates the Upanishads (foundational texts for Hinduism) "into action" is *prakriti*, which is the nature, or the "primal motive force," and there is the *atman* (the soul), or Self. When the Self identifies with nature, it merges into the *purusha*, or "knower-of-the-field." *Purusha* is the Self that pervades the universe and interacts with the material field. All devas (angelic beings) that Hindus worship embody purusha and all devis (feminine manifestation of angelic beings) embody prakriti. These complementary aspects create the necessary *tattvas* (principles) or gunas (qualities) for the creation of the universe. The ego is born from the merging of these two elements.

The ego is an instrument for action, accomplishment, and achievement in maya (the world of illusion) and is only useful in the realm of form or *samsara* (worldly existence). It is the pinstripe suit or the little black dress we wear into the world. Any form of success or achievement obtained in maya can also be destroyed. Because of the impermanence of maya, the same objects that bring us joy can also cause misery. Abiding in the Self, or the atman, is living. This is the state of "being," or "non-doing."

Being is effortless, and thus, creating from this space is effortless as well. When we meditate and repose in this space, we nurture and develop the state of consciousness where pure potentiality is possible. Develop effortlessness in life through meditation and conscious contact with Divinity.

Universal Laws

Above human-made laws are underlying universal laws. If we can learn to be in sync with these universal principles, we will live life with more ease and comfort.

It is not possible to understand the mind through the mind. We need a manual to understand how to operate certain machinery. Similarly, meditation is the experiential manual to understanding the various aspects of our existence: body, breath, memory, mind, intellect, ego, and Self. Meditation gives us access to a deeper level of understanding. From this state of awareness, we can look at the mind abstractly and detach ourselves from it. It is best to be the observer of the mind because we are not our mind or our thoughts. Perpetual thinking can be a hindrance to connecting with the Higher Self.

In twelve-step programs, emphasis is placed on action versus thought. However, when you begin to put effort into mental activity, paralysis occurs. Too much activity in the mind creates stagnation. This is a state of "analysis-paralysis."

I have a friend who continually analyzes his problems but nothing changes because he doesn't take action by making that overdue phone call or showing up to practice yoga. On one occasion he was complaining about a houseguest who had overextended his stay. When I asked him what he thought the solution was, he replied that he should call a friend to find out how to politely ask the houseguest to leave. Instead of continuing to talk about what he needed to do, I encouraged him to pick up the phone at that moment and voice his concerns to his houseguest. This was the transformational catalyst that ultimately changed his situation. It was one small action step, but it was significant enough to get the ball rolling.

Now, It's Your Turn:

Move the effort to the body. Take an action, any action. Move the energy from your head to your body.
1) Is there a task you need to be complete? Are you procrastinating something?
2) If you can't think of anything, put yourself in downward facing dog until a task comes to mind.
3) Do something. Move! Come back in twenty minutes and notice if anything has shifted.

From Thought to Action

In the awakening process, we begin to move from limited mental understanding to a level of deeper awareness and action. The atman, or Self, is stirred, and we see through the eyes that lie deep within. We move from a spectator state to an action state. If we stay in the mind, we remain in the passive spectator state: contemplating, processing, organizing, deciphering, and decoding. For true transformation to occur, we need to step on to the playing field.

This was and still is a challenge for me. By nature, I love to learn. I constantly seek out new information. But I began to realize that information is useless without application. I can intellectualize the steps and memorize the *Big Book of Alcoholics Anonymous*, but can I truly apply the program to my life? Working the sutras involves constant application. There is a reason I have gained the information and knowledge; now I must take action if I want results.

I had this issue when I was searching for an editor. I talked to many different people in the publishing world, all of whom gave me their opinion on how to select the appropriate person. Although I was being educated and gaining facts and expertise, I needed to do something. It really did not matter what I did; I just needed to find a starting point. So I emailed an author who has published books on a similar topic, and he gave me a referral. I contacted her but that editor was too busy to take on another project at that time. But she gave me another referral, and that's how I came to find the perfect editor for this book. One simple email, through a series of detours, connected me to the person I was meant to work with.

When you fertilize your inner garden through spiritual practices like yoga and meditation, love becomes your default setting. Love is inherently our default setting. Humanity will ultimately be forced to move back to its Source, and that is happening now through all the calamities in the world, such as climate change, natural disasters, and the destruction of our precious rain forest. We are literally being driven to change; Higher Consciousness is pleading to get our attention. We can continue to struggle, or we can surrender. All of us are being called, and it is possible for each of us to respond in our own way. Suffering can be human-made, but the return to love can also begin as a human-made effort.

SUTRA TWO

PRINCIPLE: Faith

DEITY: Rama

MANTRA: *Sri Rama Jayam* (Chant or write this 108 times for success in all endeavors)

(Truth is always victorious)

ASANA: *Ardha Chandrasana* (half-moon pose)

MEDITATION: Sit quietly for five minutes and repeat ten times:

"I seek to align with the power of the Divine."

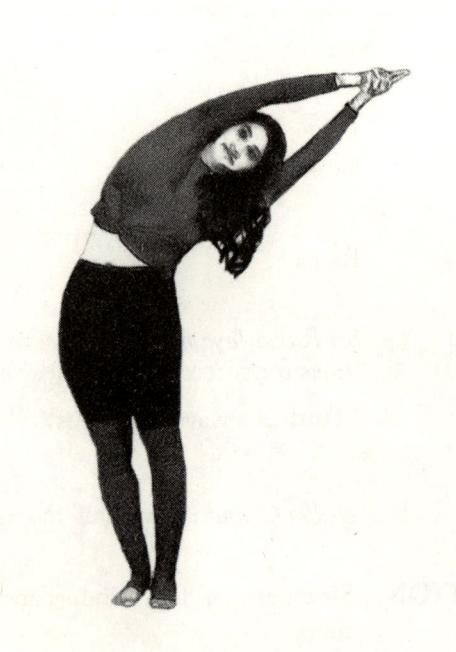

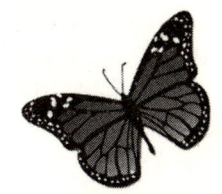

Sutra Two: Faith

Come to believe that a Power within myself could restore me to sanity

To be restored to sanity, we must face our insanity. When we come to this sutra, hopefully we recognize that our finite self, the false self, is not a very good barometer of our behavior. In our insanity, we repeat the same behaviors over and over again, expecting different results. Even more insane, we know the eventual outcome, yet we continue the behavior.

True sanity is the return to the Higher Self. When we return to the Higher Self, we are no longer driven by our ever-changing desires, running from craving to aversion. When I entered my first treatment center, I was not pleased with the facility and the daily chores we were required to complete, so I decided to leave. After relapsing, I found myself back in the same treatment center only willing to stay for thirty days of the ninety- day program. After thirty days, I left and, again, relapsed. Upon my third stay at the same treatment center, my counselor advised me to complete the full ninety days, regardless of my aversion to being confined in a treatment facility.

At that point, I had become a bit more desperate to recover after witnessing the recent overdose and death of a friend on prescription pills. Though I still had an aversion to treatment, my desire to recover became stronger and I realized that my surroundings did not matter. The return to sanity was realizing that the universe was providing me with an opportunity to recover and I could either seize that opportunity or repeat the insanity. I began to focus on what was truly important: my recovery. Once we return to our Higher Self, we gain a sense of detachment from the material world because we know, through experience from spiritual practices, that we will never find true peace and security in the material world.

Belief systems are important because they give us guidance to follow. However, belief systems also evolve or become outdated, usually in a natural progression. Once something is no longer beneficial for our highest evolution, new information arrives in a form that we are capable of digesting at that time. The Indian mystic Osho once said, "When you have a set of beliefs, drop them." The important point of Sutra Two is to be open-minded.

Being raised in Hindu culture, I was taught to embrace all faiths and find wisdom in all holy texts. The underlying message is the same; only the interpretation changes. If we expose ourselves to as many different concepts as possible, we gain the ability to understand not only ourselves, but also the world in various ways. As our understanding and awareness grow deeper, we are able to connect to other people on a number of levels. It is like being fluent in several languages.

When we understand a thought or belief system, we can utilize it for our greatest good and part with it when necessary. Treat every belief as a guest; invite them all in. Be open to the vast amount of knowledge in the world. Consider nutrients from food. Amino acids do not change, but the sources from which we derive them do. If we understand this, we can feast abundantly.

Faith + Action

There is a saying in twelve-step programs: "Faith without works is dead." I once sat in a *homa puja*, a Hindu prayer ritual of honor and worship, at a temple in Chicago and I was amazed at the amount of faith I witnessed. I began to wonder how much action followed this overwhelming display of faith. Faith and prayer are beautiful, but we cannot expect the Divine to make house calls. Action rewards prayer and faith with a new reality.

For most of my life, I knew in my heart that I would write a book. In fact, at the age of six, my parents bought me a small, old-fashioned typewriter and I would type stories, illustrated with Mickey Mouse stickers. Writing was an innate gift from the beginning. I always carried the thought in my head that I should write a book. But nothing was happening because it remained merely a thought, a wish, an empty dream. I had to take action and put pen to paper. When I took the smallest action, the universe supported me and propelled my journey forward.

When we couple faith with action, we often experience synchronicity, or so-called "coincidences." When faith is strong, even small steps produce extraordinary experiences. Moving from faith to manifestation occurs through *sankalpa,* or intention. When I have a sankalpa and know that it is aligned with universal law, action becomes effortless because the idea is fully supported. Intention requires faith because you are setting a goal without limiting the parameters under which you want that goal to be met.

For example, the year I set the intention to actually write this book, I made a list of all the goals I wanted to achieve and one of those goals was to finish my graduate education. During my active addiction, my life had become too chaotic to finish my master's degree in clinical psychology. I was popping Vicodin all day in class. Eventually, the pills became my priority and I took a leave of absence from school.

Seven years later, I decided that I wanted to finish school. I clearly wrote on a piece of paper, "I want to study more and finish school." I was open to how the universe would guide me to do this. The intention was set; now it was just a matter of being open to accepting the opportunities placed in my path. After taking some action steps and doing the research, I found a master's-track program in addictions counseling being offered at a small school close to where I was living at the time. All my graduate coursework transferred into this program. It was a perfect match! I could never have conjured up this plan, but the universe surely could.

This is a prime example of setting an intention, exploring your options through action, and then being open to receiving the blessings of your intention. You trust the universe to find the best possible way to deliver. You trust the process and let go as the results fall into place. As you continually do this and witness the Divine co-creating with you, your faith in the Divine increases and you begin to rely on this Power to guide and direct you in your life. You begin to realize that you no longer feel the need for control. You can become a witness to your own life. When you let go and let the universe work its magic, a sense of relief suffuses your being.

Now, It's Your Turn:
1) Find a piece of paper and write down one goal you want to accomplish.
2) Write with confidence that your goal will be fulfilled.
3) After you write this goal down, say it out loud so the universe hears you! Speak with conviction. Transfer it from the mind into *akasha* (space).
4) Next, take one action step to move yourself closer to this goal. Google it, make a phone call, or email someone who will provide you with more information.
5) Research and receive!

Here are a few examples:

Write: "I want to get in shape."

Say It: "I am getting in shape" (in the present tense–this moment is all there is!).

Action Step: Find and join a local gym or call a friend and set up weekly running dates. (It always helps to get others working with you to achieve your goal!)

Write: "I want to learn to speak another language."

Say It: "I am learning to speak French."

Action Step: Find an online language-immersion course or travel to your nearest library and pick up an introductory book on the French language. Ready, set, move! Your life is waiting!

When we apply our knowledge, we become the master of our own destiny. Knowledge, application, and repetition essentially form our character. We are molding ourselves into who we want to become. Thus, there is a difference between understanding something and embodying something.

Self-Mastery

Our goal in life is self-mastery. We begin by learning something, mastering it, then embodying it. If you want to really understand and benefit from yoga, embody it; become yoga. *Yoga* simply means "union." Unify with everything. Spiritual practices, like yoga, will become a way of life when you embody their virtues. Any practice can be done from this "yogic" mind-set, even writing. For me, writing is a matter of unifying creativity, self-exploration, and personal experience. The audience I write for is myself.

When you embody knowledge, your life becomes a flow. You no longer question situations. You simply move through them, take in life's nutrients, and discard the pulp or filler. The external world is the world of lack and limitation. The internal world is where true wealth resides. Once you awaken to this truth, you live your life on a different dimension. When you learn to "flow" through life, you become more connected to your dharma, or purpose, here on the physical plane.

The questions are these: How long do you want to wait until you discover what your purpose is? Are you satisfied with your level of awareness or just comfortable living in ignorance? Does your ego fear change because you feel as though you may lose something? I pray to abandon ideas and beliefs that no longer serve my highest good. I pray to gain what will nourish my spirit and aid me in progressing toward liberation.

In hindsight, it did not matter whether I went to AA, NA, CA (Cocaine Anonymous), or PA (Pills Anonymous). The ultimate gifts were the Twelve Sutras and recovery. There are many paths. Choose one and follow it wholeheartedly. Bring your awareness into every moment. I adamantly respect all religions because truth is universal.

I once asked a friend what the basis of Catholicism is and what a rosary represents. As she explained her understanding of this faith, her eyes lit up and she exuded enthusiasm. I was listening to music. Faith is seeing without sight, a sense of knowing. It is a feeling that something exists beyond our limited senses.

The "power" greater than ourselves is our Self, or atman. When we turn our ego over to the pure consciousness of which it was born, we gain our real power. So, in this sense, the power we seek is already within us. Swami Chinmayananda notes, "The individual is nothing but the Supreme itself, the individual has arisen from It, exists in It, and merges back into It. This ego-center has thus been created certainly out of the Atman, but at the same time, the ego has not got any independent existence apart from the Divine spark, our own Self."[1]

The ego is to the atman, our soul, what a shadow is to a person. The ego is part of the *atman* but has no separate identity, power, or value unless we strengthen its identity. We control the intensity of our ego. Many people talk about getting rid of their ego. Don't try to rid yourself of your ego: The more you try, the stronger it will grow. Whatever you focus your attention on will grow. Acknowledge your ego when it shows up in your consciousness, because without it you would not be able to return to your true Self. The ego structure allows for the return or completion of pravritti (outward-directed action) back to nivritti (inward-directed action). If you observe emotional people, they are continually identifying with their fleeting thoughts. The goal is to return to a place that is solid and unshakable through any storm.

When I began working Sutra Two, I only had a few weeks abstinent from drugs and alcohol. I was going through withdrawal and would burst out into tears at the most inopportune moments. I was overwhelmed with fear and anxiety. All the emotions I had stuffed down with drugs were starting to come to the surface. I recall days when the most I could do for the day was take a shower. I had little faith in myself, let alone an unknown "Power" that was supposed to magically cure me.

Since I had little understanding of a Higher Power, I relied heavily on the Pills Anonymous (PA) and Narcotics Anonymous (NA) fellowships in 2012. My recovery companions were my pillars of strength. I suppose they were my Higher Power in the beginning. I went to two meetings a week regularly for the first few months of my recovery. Some days, I literally felt carried by the women in the fellowship.

I remember one woman in PA saying, "I'm strong today, so I can be there for you. When you are strong, you will be there for me. And that's how this thing works." That same woman called me six months later after her husband committed suicide; she was hysterical. She was right; I was strong that day and could be there as a support for her. Community support is vital in recovery, especially from those who have gone through similar experiences.

In 12-Step programs, people often refer to God as "Group of Drunks," because some struggle with a concept of a Higher Power. The group becomes the surrogate Higher Power. I was so beat down in early recovery that I struggled to really believe there was a Higher Power out there, and that this "Power" was paying attention to me. For the time being, the PA and NA fellowships worked as my Higher Power. Now I can see that my Higher Power was working through these people and was there all along. Through spiritual practices (yoga, meditation, and Sudarshan Kriya), I began to feel that this Power and my Self were not that different from one another. I began to feel this Power working through me, as if I were the instrument.

The Source of Our Power

So, in Sutra Two, we seek power from our Higher Self. Our finite self, or ego, is powerless, but our Higher Consciousness is immeasurably powerful. Higher Consciousness is always accessible and, once we access it, there are no limitations to our power. This step states *come to believe,* but we must go beyond belief straight to faith, or *sraddha*. Sutra Two is all about faith. The only thing that can shake faith is doubt, and doubt is a subtle form of fear, which is not of our true nature and does not really exist.

In the Hindu epic *Ramayana*, the avatar Rama goes on a long and arduous journey to save his wife, Sita, from the grips of Ravana, the evil monarch of Lanka. Initially, Rama does not know if Sita has been killed by Ravana, but he has faith that she is alive and that he will find her. With Hanuman's help, Rama carries out his dharma and eventually finds Sita and saves her.

Sita remained faithful to Rama, ignoring Ravana's temptations. Despite opposition from the people of the land, Rama eventually accepted Sita back and restored her rightly seat as queen. Rama was able to restore virtue and order; his rule ushered in a golden age. Another ending of this myth claims Sita returned to mother earth. Sita exuded bravery, keeping her faith in Rama, and in the end, her faith to the Source (mother earth), from where all things originate. Rama eventually abandoned Sita to please the people of his kingdom, Ayodhya, however, legend has it that Rama and Sita were once again reunited in the eternal realm. Faith is knowing beyond what is known, despite any apparent circumstances. The story of Sita and Rama exemplifies faith and love.

So when our mind clings to the illusion of fear, we move away from our center, which is love. This is where faith dwells. So what should we have faith in? Have faith in your light, in your essence, which is love. Transcend even the idea of darkness. Go beyond all illusion to truth.

Swami Chinmayananda elaborates:

"Even to say that there is darkness, we must be conscious of it. The "light" of awareness is so subtle and Absolute that it illumines not only the various sources of light in the world, but also the experience of darkness itself. That which illumines both light and darkness must be a factor that transcends both these experiences."[2]

In yoga, *ardha chandrasana*, or half-moon pose, is symbolic of the golden moon avatar. The light from the moon illuminates the dark sky at night. Without the moonlight, there would be complete darkness. But it is the speck of light in the midst of darkness that enables us to see. That is faith; the speck of light that enables us to see. Rama used this light to see and was eventually reunited with his true love.

A belief is simply a group of organized thoughts, but there is no evidence outside your thoughts to prove that your beliefs are true. The vast amount of knowledge in this world derives from many different sources. Once you are on a spiritual path, you understand the wisdom in each tradition and that all sources of knowledge eventually merge into one.

When I was in graduate school, I was taking a postmodernist psychology class and we were giving presentations on different theoretical orientations. It was interesting to watch the narrative-therapy people defend their belief system and the existential group discuss the here and now. My presentation was on Jung and how the concepts of the anima and animus compared to Hindu god/goddess mythology. Our teacher just sat back and laughed. He said, "These are all just gimmicks!"

It is as though our thoughts need a vessel, and a belief system is that vessel. But the questions are these: What do we do with this vessel? What becomes of it? Some of us cling to it until it no longer serves us except as a crutch because we don't know how to operate without it. It makes up so much of who we are that if we were to lose it, we would feel as if we had lost our very selves.

But how can you be confined to one set of thoughts? Are you not curious about others? I am a student of Vedanta, yet I choose to explore all religions. A belief or thought system can often be seen as a religion. It may direct you on a certain path, but it may also be a barrier to your growth.

SUTRA THREE

DEITY: Dattatreya

PRINCIPLE: Willingness

MANTRA: *Shri Gurudev Datta*
(One who provides frequencies of divine consciousness)

ASANA: *Kakasana* (crow pose)

MEDITATION: Sit quietly for five minutes and repeat ten times:

"Hand in hand, will as One, I prevail and overcome."

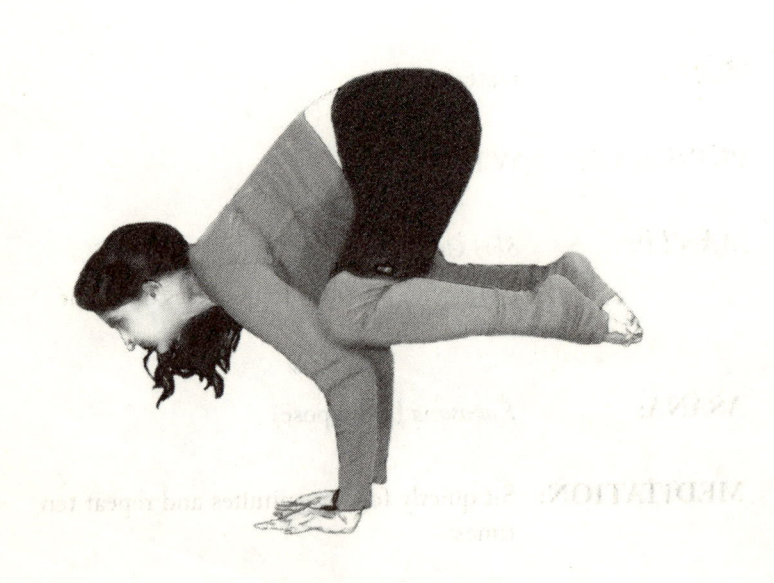

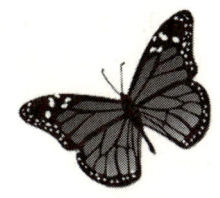

Sutra Three: Willingness

Make a decision to align my will and life with the Divine, as I understand the Divine

In Alcoholics Anonymous, part of Step 3 reads, "turn my will and life over," which to me meant, "give all my burdens to the Higher Power." My sponsor at the time noted that this step required me to surrender all my fears, worries, and concerns to the "care of the Divine," as the rest of the step states. A question arose in my mind: Why is this Power big enough to handle my addiction, but not my depression? It made absolutely no sense to me. So, as my willingness to lean on this Power grew, I took a risk and started weaning myself off my psychotropic medications, which was not easy, but I had tools (yoga, meditation, SKY) to aid in the uncomfortable process.

I remember feeling suicidal at times through this weaning off process. After all, my brain was going through massive neurological changes; the neurotransmitters were imbalanced. Yet, I accepted these symptoms were part of the recovery process and stayed willing to endure it by taking necessary action. I trusted my Higher Power and my own intuition. In essence, through SKY and meditation, the universe's will (plan) aligned with my will. Despite the conflicting advice I received from medical professionals, who were strongly opposed to me going off the meds, which included my parents, both allopathic doctors, I took the risk and "made a decision to align my will and life with the Divine." It was at this point that I began researching Ayurveda and found an Ayurvedic practitioner who guided me. I began implementing Ayurvedic principles into my lifestyle and these treatments helped immensely, expediting the detox process.

Let's consider our "will." Our will is the ego-center. In twelve-step programs, many people ask this question: "How do I know if it's God's will or my will?"

I struggled with this for some time because I was trying to understand my will using my limited mental faculties. Through spiritual practice and meditation, I developed an internal-consciousness or tuning to the Higher Self. In meditation, as you attune yourself to Divinity, you cultivate your intuition. Then your will becomes universal will; the two wills align. The ego-center or individualized identity merges back into the Self, or *atman*.

Keep in mind that there is a difference between having an idea of Divinity and having an experience of Divinity. Turning your will over to the care of an idea is different from turning your will over to a Higher Power. An idea is merely a construct of the mind. When the life force, or *prana*, filters through the mind, it expresses itself as the individualized ego-center. The sense of ego in Vedanta is called the *jeeva*. Swami Chinmayananda elaborates:

"The individual Life, the *Prana*, is but the reflection of Pure Consciousness in our mind and intellect. Consciousness or awareness, when It works through the "flow of thoughts"–the mind–expresses Itself in a "reflection" which is the ego-centric personality that we come to recognize almost always as ourselves.[1]"

So, in essence, Divinity cannot be logically understood. An idea can be understood in an individual's subjective mind, but an energy of consciousness can only be experienced. This experience of Higher-consciousness is illustrated beautifully in the story of Shams and Rumi:

"Who is greater, the prophet Mohammed or the great teacher Betsami? Without hesitation Rumi answered, 'Of course, the prophet Mohammed.'

Shams had to see what Rumi was made of, so he took his questioning one step further. "Betsami, the distinguished teacher, said, 'I am great because God is within me,' whereas Mohammed said, 'God is great in His infinite mercy.' How would you explain this?"

Overcome by the personal significance of this question, Rumi fell to his knees. Shams had just unlocked a door deep within Rumi's soul. Even though Betsami was considered one of the greatest scholars of his time, Rumi found little solace in his holy books. He had settled into life as a teacher but felt spiritually unfulfilled. Finding Shams was unexpected and astonishing. In that instant Rumi knew that no book could teach him what his soul could."[2]

A Course in Miracles states that "We are an idea in the mind of God."[3] The jeeva, or ego, is a reflection of the atman, which comes from the reflecting mechanism, the mind. The mind in this respect is but a tool. It is like a film projector that shows a movie. The roll of film contains the same scenes as what actually gets depicted on the screen. In following the Twelve-Sutras, we aim to be free of resentments, ill will, and negativity. The mind needs to be polished and clean to clearly reflect the atman. This is why we continually take inventory in the fourth and tenth sutras.

A Course in Miracles goes on to state, "Ideas leave not their source."[4] The jeeva is born from the atman, so there is only one original source of existence or consciousness but when this consciousness is filtered or projected through the mind, it presents itself as the individualized body–the ego (jeeva). What we consider our separate, individualized self is not actually its own identity. The problem arises when we understand this persona to be who we truly are. Our vision becomes distorted.

Detours from Our Dharma

In Hindu thought, the ego's propensity to vacillate from craving to aversion and to fuel desire causes the cycle of rebirth. We are all born in human form to serve in some capacity, to fulfill our dharma. But when we arrive on earth, our agenda changes. In the allure of maya, illusion sways us from our earthly calling and we succumb to the desires of the ego. We take detours on our path.

For example, in 2006, I entered a twelve-step program, which initially helped me get sober. Once I began to accrue consecutive days of sobriety and work the twelve steps, my life started to fall into place and I was accepted into a graduate clinical psychology program. It was my dharmic destiny to pursue higher studies. But the temptation of maya prevailed and I became distracted by my involvement in a relationship with another individual in recovery. Eventually, the relationship and my failure to stay on my path triggered a relapse and I was back to square one. We are on a continuous journey of learning. Like a small child who learns after learns his lessons by getting scolded, we will continue to suffer blows from maya until we understand that the nature of maya is deceptive.

When we are filled with the positive vibrations of Higher Consciousness, we desire very little because we know we already possess everything we need. The guru Sri Sri Ravi Shankar emphasizes that when you are on the spiritual path, you walk like a king because you have everything you need to flourish. When you walk with the confidence of a king or queen, you embody that regal vibration and your world becomes a magical kingdom.

We live on a physical plane and in order to function in the world of form, we must have sensory perception. Our essence is the atman but our functional component is the ego, or jeeva. Ego, which is born from atman, has no individualized identity. However, ego tends to identify as Self and act as though it were separate from its origin. The small mind forgets it is part of the large mind. When we identify with mind and ego, we get lost in cravings, desires, and the accumulation of material things. According to Swami Chinmayananda:

"The Self identifying with the gross body expresses itself as the perceiver and thereafter recognizes the world of objects as being other than itself. Expressing through the physical body and its sense organs, the Jeeva gathers its quota of pleasures by indulging in sense objects."[5]

The function of the ego is described in this analogy in *Vedanta: The Science of Life:*

"The man dwells in his house and goes out daily into the world to strive for his livelihood. After earning his means of existence, he returns home to enjoy what he has earned and to rest a while. Rested and refreshed under the scrutiny of his house, he moves out again the following day, full of energy, to meet the challenges of the new day. In the same way, the ego moves out of the physical body to contact the sense objects and returns to it to savor its joys and sorrows."[6]

When you experience joy from multiple sources, your ego no longer seeks to cling to the object it believes is solely responsible for your joy. For many years, I believed that the source of my joy was found in a relationship. I would meet someone and the first three months would be complete bliss. However, I discovered that this infatuation and attachment are short-lived. Ultimately, the initial source of joy loses its appeal and we move on to the next desire. The cyclic nature of attachment causes suffering and distorts the experience of true joy.

Joy and love are abundant and can be manifested in any situation. They have no boundaries or limitations because the Source is infinite. Our nature is divine love and every relationship we are in—romantic or platonic—is an exchange of this one love. This is true Power and you have the capability to tap into this infinite reservoir with every human interaction. This was the realization I needed to understand—that I didn't need to be in a romantic relationship to experience love. When you see that the love you seek is ever-present in all forms, you do not become attached to a specific type of packaging.

What you believe to be true is your truth. If you believe you are a successful author, you will be. If you believe life is struggle, it will be. In yoga, *kakasana* is also known as crow pose. Have you ever watched a group of crows ganging up with one another and chasing out birds much bigger than they are? Crows possess a personal willpower. They do not know their own size in relation to the other birds, but that does not limit their desire for their prey.

Now, It's Your Turn:

Challenge a limiting belief.
1) Think of one dominating belief you hold to be true about yourself. For example, "I'm not qualified to get that job." "I'm not attractive enough for that person."
2) Now, rephrase that belief (say it out loud, into akasha): "I'm qualified, and worthy of _____." (Fill in the blank.)
3) It's up to you. How much love and abundance are you ready for? If you believe it, you will see it!

Fear versus Love

Our ego would like us to dwell in these lower-frequency thoughts because the ego wants us to choose fear. But when we become dedicated to knowing ourselves, we find that our "real" authentic Self is only love. The more we learn to operate from our Higher Self and positive frequencies, the easier it is to maneuver through life on the "love" vibration. Invest in yourself and do only good for yourself. Nurture yourself with love.

In a state of equanimity, where there is neither craving nor aversion, the ego becomes dormant and we do not fall prey to the feverish wants and demands the ego is notorious for. The terminology in the world of recovery refers to the "ism." The ism, or I, self, and me, can only be eradicated by shifting our thinking to something outside ourselves. The *Big Book of Alcoholics Anonymous* makes reference to this "constant thought of others."[7] Cultivating a sense of selflessness is essential to eradicating this tendency among addicted individuals toward self-obsession, or the focus on asmita.

The ego expresses constant wants and desires, with an underlying need to gratify the self in some manner. What we desire—the addictive substance—is not actually the problem. The pills were not my problem; it was my desire for them. The unsettling feverishness, craving, or mental obsession—that is the root of our problem. When we are in a state of equanimity, we feel contentment and stability within. Whether our desire or craving is fulfilled becomes irrelevant because we remain content in its absence. A strength resides within us that has no need. It is perfectly whole and content; this is the residence of our solace.

When we become centered and grounded within ourselves, our attachments to worldly objects dissolve and the need to acquire or gain vanishes. When we are fully absorbed in this state, the ego takes a back seat. Dattatreya is considered by Hindus to be an incarnation of the divine trinity: Brahma, Vishnu, and Shiva. Dattatreya left home at an early age to wander in search of the Absolute, or Supreme. This willingness to explore the truth is necessary for spiritual gain in recovery.

Dattatreya was first considered a "Lord of Yoga," with siddhis, or inherent gifts. The word Datta means "Given," Datta is called so because the divine trinity have "given" themselves in the form of a son to the sage couple Atri and Anasuya. He is the son of Atri, hence the name "Atreya." Dattatreya is usually depicted with three heads (Brahma, Vishnu, Shiva), representing the past, present, and future. We cannot change our past, but we can accept the present and live fully in this moment, paving the way for a bright future. To free himself from all worldly attachments, Dattatreya dove into a lake where he stayed for many years; he chose to journey into the unknown, beyond the fearful limitations of the mortal mind.

The ego's need to acquire and accumulate has no effect on us. Who we are will remain constant through material losses and gains. The world is rajasic; that is, it functions via activity. The collective egoic mind wants to accumulate worldly objects This is the reason for economic disparity. This need for more stems from an innate feeling of lack that gets projected into the world; this then reverberates through our life to our detriment. The only way to free ourselves from the collective bondage perpetuated by society is to remain grounded within ourselves and to know that our spiritual essence is abundance.

Nourishing the Soul

Spiritual nourishment is essential. Without food, we starve. Similarly, without divine nourishment, our system becomes depleted of vital nutrients needed to sustain our true essence and strength. In contemporary society, this daily spiritual maintenance is crucial.

We must continually stay connected to our Source. The poverty we see across the world is a reflection of our spiritual poverty. In order to uplift the world, we must uplift our sattvic nature. When we become more sattvic (that is, filled with goodness), the world as a whole will become more sattvic. In Hindu philosophy, sattvic represents purity, serenity, and forgiveness. These are qualities that our world clearly needs more of. As sattva increases, the moral standards of society will increase. Moving away from rajas (mindless activity), toward sattva (goodness and purity), is a step toward liberation. A sattvic mind frees us from rajasic, egoic desires. Moving away from the focus on self to the focus on service, or *seva*, is the natural direction of spiritual evolution.

SUTRA FOUR

DEITY: Shiva

PRINCIPLE: Courage

MANTRA: *Om Namah Shivaya*

Om Namah Shivaya quells the instinct, cuts through the steel bands, and turns this intellect within and on itself, to face itself and see its ignorance. This mantra is life, action, and love, and with each repetition wisdom bursts forth from within.

ASANA: *Natarajasana* (dancing Shiva)

MEDITATION: Sit in a quiet spot for five minutes. Repeat silently ten times with your eyes closed:

"With courage at last, I release my past."

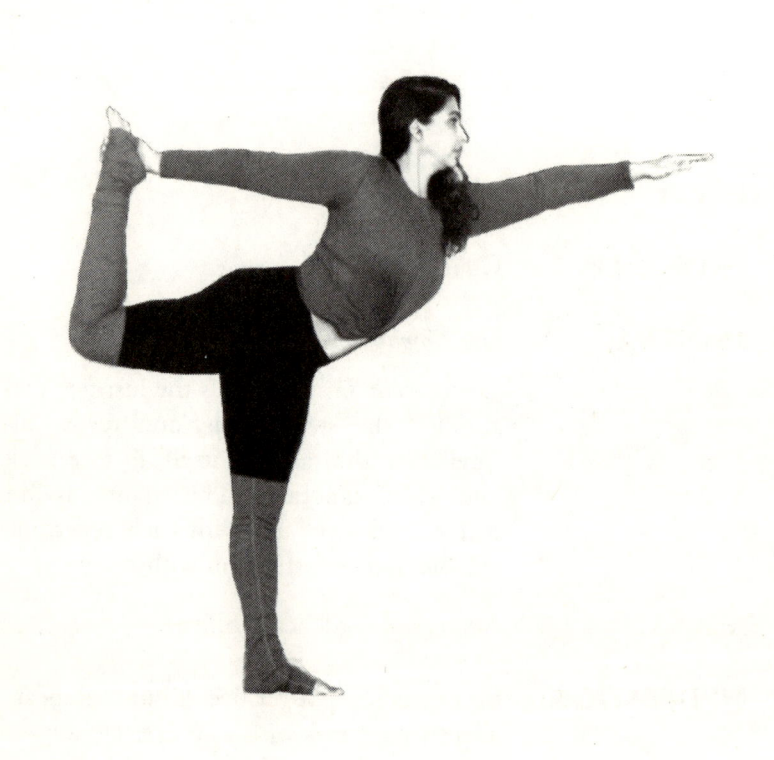

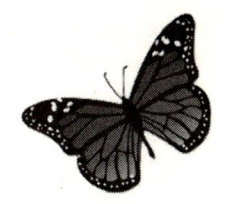

Sutra Four: Courage

*Make a fearless and loving
moral inventory of myself*

In active addiction, fears and resentments seem to be the common denominator for much of our struggle. Resentments are thoughts about the past; they are over, gone, done. Other than bringing them into our consciousness through rumination, they do not exist. So when you are experiencing a resentful thought, observe that your mind is in the past. Take action and consciously move forward.

When we dwell on the past, we diminish our ability to stay focused on the present moment and oftentimes experience discomfort or "dis-ease." Why spend time analyzing something that does not exist? It does not serve us, nor does it serve the Divine. There is work to be done in this moment. Be present; uplift those around you. When you come to realize this is your sole purpose here, you will no longer choose resentment, anger, or remorse. When you come to understand dharma and accept your responsibility, you will use time more effectively.

At times, fear overwhelms me. Fear appears to exist, but it is only an illusion, a projection of the mind. So if you are fearful, you have bought into the illusion. Proceed with caution because what you fear becomes charged and manifests in various ways. Conversely, what you have faith in, you will attract. Thoughts initiate our circumstances, so give energy to kind, loving thoughts and kindness and love will manifest in your life. When your thoughts and actions are focused on service and love, the universe responds with gratitude because you are in alignment with the higher cause.

I have much admiration for Marianne Williamson's work. When I interned for her, all my energy was directed toward carrying her vision into the larger world and sharing her message with others. The payoff was the high I experienced being of service, sharing her wisdom, and seeing the transformation in others. What a joy to see people realize their divinity!

Leave room for all the ways the universe will bring to fruition your deepest intentions. Continue to plant seeds, put out the energy you want to receive. Don't just plant a garden; cultivate a plantation and harvest a multitude of possibilities. Remember that you are not the doer. When we get lost in "doing," we move away from "being." Be a clear channel for the Divine to shower you with the love and abundance that are your due. The easiest way for the universe to provide this abundance is to clear your channel of past karma. So let's look at karma.

How Karma Dovetails with Recovery

Karma means "action." On some level, the Twelve Sutras can make us aware of our habitual behaviors, or actions, which create our karma. Karma has also been accumulated from past lives and past impressions called *samskaras*. Dr. Brian Weiss, psychotherapist and past life regression expert, comments, "Sometimes the tendency toward substance abuse itself is one that has been carried over from previous lifetimes."[1] Some of this karmic residue can only be eliminated by cultivating a state of awareness beyond the mind and intellect.

Karma may begin at the level of thought. When we discipline our mind, we can choose positive thoughts more often, which lead to positive actions. But here again, we find that we will not be able to manipulate the mind through the mind. In a sense, we need to observe the mind from a distance in order to exercise control over it.

Swami Chinmayananda states, "Thoughts classified and marshaled through consistent reflection (*mananam*) order the mind into a definite pattern, and this determines the texture, efficiency, sincerity, and quality of actions. Thought tracks in the mind ramble into actions. Thus, karma evolves out of the thought-patterns in ourselves."[2]

Experiences in our current life and from our past lives create *samskaras*, or impressions. These impressions precipitate feelings that generate desire. The person with an addiction tends to cling to feelings and act according to cravings or aversions. When we feel good, we want to feel better; when we feel bad, we want to feel good.

For years, I used drugs to suppress painful emotions. In the early days of my recovery, I experienced an emotional detoxification. I would call my sponsor on the phone every day, emotionally distraught, and her response was always the same, "Feelings are not facts." We are always looking for ways to maintain bliss, induced by the drug or from a natural high. So, in order to move toward a healthy, balanced state of mind, body, and emotional equilibrium, we must eliminate some of these negative *samskaras* and stop creating dissonance.

In recovery, *hitting rock bottom* means we can no longer run from our own karma. The universe has put us in a situation that forces us to face our past. If we want to evolve and progress on the spiritual path, we must confront and eliminate negative karma from our present and past lives.

In Sutra Four, we take an honest look at our karmic deficits. The cycle of karma and attachment keeps us bound to the world of form. When we accumulate karma of merit, or positive karma, this will translate into the peace we experience in the afterlife. Once that merit expires, we come back to the earth to work again and the cycle of life and death continues. There is no evolution in maya; the world of form has limitations. We must strive to dwell in the realm of supreme infinite consciousness; only from this place is self-realization possible. Sutra Four is the beginning of the disintegration of the false self. We are bringing the darkness into light. We become aware of the ego's propensity to keep us trapped in fear, and we seek to align ourselves with our inner guru.

From Inertia to Action

At Sutra Four, we invoke Shiva. Shiva is the deity of dissolution and transformation. In Sutras One through Three, we are still in a tamasic state (a state of darkness) and we want to move toward the rajasic state and eventually into a sattvic state. So we invoke Shiva, the lord of dissolution, to clear away an inert state of being and move into an active state of mind. All that begins must end and all that is created is eventually destroyed. Shiva represents the natural force of destruction and transformation within nature. Without clearing out the old, creation cannot occur. Endings can require courage—destruction may not always seem pleasant. Shiva has three eyes symbolizing the sun, the moon, and fire, the three sources of illumination. Using the outer and inner sources of light, we garner our courage and move ahead fearlessly.

When we make our karmic inventory, we get a glimpse of our past. It is natural to feel strong emotions as we work through this Sutra. Those close to us may notice when we work on fourth-sutra inventory, because the fourth sutra is the first of the cleansing and release sutras. We feel uncomfortable when we are reminded of our past behaviors while in a tamasic state of mind. This is where we can apply acceptance and encourage ourselves to continue moving forward toward liberation and freedom.

I had several resentments toward my family, but when I sat down and wrote my fourth-sutra inventory, I saw the part I had played in each situation. I had a resentment toward my mother; however, I had stolen money from her bank account to buy drugs at one point. It was difficult to look at the evidence but, deep within, I knew that my behavior was not a reflection of who I truly was. I accepted that I had made mistakes, but more important, I had firmly resolved to atone for those mistakes because freedom from my past was crucial to becoming the person I was destined to be. We need to make a clearing for our extraordinary nature to flourish.

Sutra Four is pivotal because it begins the tamasic clarifying and cleansing process. Many people in recovery get to Sutra Three and stop. Why? Because they must be willing to endure temporary discomfort in Sutra Four. However, we have to push forward with faith and trust in the process. Try to set aside a day or a block of time to start the fourth sutra. I would recommend being as thorough as possible, but do not become obsessed with perfecting it. You will complete other fourth sutras later in life and you can always maintain this practice with a daily tenth sutra.

Now, It's Your Turn:

Make your columnized lists as follows:
1) Resentment (person, place, thing, organization):
2) Cause of resentment:
3) What was my motivation, or what did I believe, that led me to act as I did in these situations?
4) Area of Life Affected (personal relationships, ambition, security, financial):
5) My Part (character defects):

Now answer these questions:
1) How has "My Part" contributed to these resentments?
2) How have my resentments affected my relationships with myself, with others, and with my Higher Power?

Make as thorough a list as possible. Become aware if you begin to judge yourself (the ego will attempt to defeat you before you begin). Keep going! Become the lion!

In the fourth sutra, we begin to acknowledge the past with the intention of correcting our karma; this enables us to move forward. The yoga asana called *natarajasana*, dancing Shiva, represents this process. Balancing on one leg, our arm grasps the other leg from behind, yet the chest is upright and one arm extends forward. This is symbolic of the acknowledgment of the past with the resolve and courage to move forward. Often in a yoga practice, this is one of the most difficult postures because it requires so much tenacity and endurance. It is a highly skilled posture that challenges your comfort zone.

The *Narcotics Anonymous* textbook states, "Courage is demonstrated not by the lack of fear, but by the actions we take in spite of the fear."[3] Our ultimate fear is the lack of faith in ourselves and our own power. In Sutra Four, we demonstrate courage by taking action. We become the lion in Sutras Four through Nine. We have reached the point of complete surrender and now we morph into the warrior who must enter the battlefield. But we are armed with the faith that we have been drafted by the Divine.

In India, the *Kshatriyas* were originally the soldiers. Their dharma was to protect the good of the world through battle. In Sutra Four, we begin to take action, or pravritti, in much the same way that the Kshatriyas took to the battlefield.

This is similar to the epic, the *Mahabharata*. In the *Mahabharata*, before the start of such a war being waged by the Kshatriya Pandavas, their main warrior Arjuna develops a dilemma: Arjuna has surrendered to Krishna, his divine Self, but to fulfill his dharma he must wage war against his own cousins. Arjuna is very hesitant to fight his own kin and to kill another human, especially his own family. Symbolically, Arjuna's cousins, the *Kauravas*, represent the desires that cause us to forget our dharma and get lost in the world of ego and form.

Swami Chidbhavananda quotes from the Bhagavad Gita: "In the Bhagavad Gita, Arjuna asks Krishna, 'Under what compulsion does a man commit sin, in spite of himself, and driven, as it were, by force?' Krishna replies, 'It is desire, it is wrath, which springs from rajas.'"[4]

Arjuna eventually knows that as a warrior, fighting is his duty, so he must follow through. But he is never alone because Lord Krishna is always with him. Therefore, his action becomes *Karma Yoga*—when work is done without any desire for personal gain. The actions you take are aligned with those that God wants you to take.

From Spiritual Bondage to Liberation

In Sutra Four, we start digging to find where our false self has wreaked havoc. In the *Big Book of Alcoholics Anonymous*, this is referred to as, "clearing away the wreckage of our past." We are moving from spiritual bondage to spiritual liberation and beginning the process of forgiveness. Sutra Four takes courage, tenacity, and perseverance.

When we begin Sutra Four, hopefully we are aware that it no longer serves us or this world to act in accordance with the ego and maintain the illusion that our finite selves have any authority. It starts to become evident that we must make some changes after we see the part we have played in our own circumstances. While writing my fourth sutra, I began to see a recurring character defect: selfishness.

The ego always acts to preserve itself, even if it affects another person adversely. I bore a huge resentment against the district attorney who wanted to sentence me to four months in jail after I received a felony DUI. I was outraged at the severity of this punishment. But after writing out my inventory, I saw that the punishment was appropriate for hitting a vehicle with two passengers inside. Actually, I had gotten off fairly easy. I remember the words of a woman in my jail cell the night I was arrested: "You are lucky you didn't kill anyone. You would be doing life in prison."

After Sutra Two, I captured a glimpse of my insanity, based on actions repetitively propelled by self-will. In my case, the results were absolute self-will unhinged.

Pursuing the fourth sutra, by writing a moral inventory, exposes the ego. We begin to separate our true Self from the egoic structure that has been built around it. Unless we expose the false self, we never see the truth. The entire process of twelve-sutra work is designed to deepen our relationship with our Higher Self, which is ultimately our "Higher Power." Before you begin work on this sutra, keep in mind that you are not inherently bad. You were operating from your level of awareness at that time, which was tamasic, dull, and cloudy. Do not crucify yourself. You are not your past. As you move forward in recovery and work the remaining sutras, more will be revealed, and your true nature will shine through. We are raising the curtains so the sun can illuminate our true Self.

Banishing Resentment, Anger, and Ill Will

Removing resentment, anger, and ill will from the mind is crucial on the spiritual path of recovery. When anger and hostility dominate the mind, people tend to project that into society. A peace agreement between countries begins with a peace agreement within oneself. External reality is always a reflection of inner harmony or disharmony.

The purpose of this moral inventory is to cleanse the mind of negative thoughts, which lead to negative feelings, which are then expressed by negative actions. When we write down our resentments, we release the energy and space they occupy in our mind. A dear sponsor once told me, "Those resentments are living rent-free in your mind." We also look at how we can take responsibility and own "our part," compassionately, without condemning ourselves for our past. We must keep in mind that our actions in the past were set in motion from a lower level of consciousness. As we deepen our awareness, we begin to live our lives more authentically and genuinely. Sutra Four enables us to recognize who we really are and the essence of our true nature.

When we write our inventory in the fourth step, we see how the small mind—the mind associated with worldly objects and illusion—has clouded our judgment and how this has brought about suffering in our lives. Although we live in this world of form, it is important not to be "of" the world of form. The lotus flower sits above the water with its roots anchored in the mud. We must remain above the mud of maya.

To begin to move into a sattvic state and utilize the "pure" mind, or pure consciousness, which is our essence, we must cleanse and release whatever no longer serves our higher evolution or our goal of liberation. We each need to liberate our mind, which enables us to liberate our Self. Releasing and consciously letting go of the past is the beginning of this freedom. A thorough inventory allows for more cleansing, which inevitably makes space for thoughts and actions that serve our highest and greatest good. Without commitment to this Sutra, little transformation is possible.

SUTRA FIVE

DEITY: Parvati

PRINCIPLE: Trust

MANTRA: *Annapurne Shankar Prane Parvati Namostute*
(Salutations to the provider who delivers the Shiva Shakti)

ASANA: *Sirsasana* (headstand)

MEDITATION: Sit in a quiet spot. Close your eyes and repeat ten times silently:

"Everything I see, I trust to be, the highest for me."

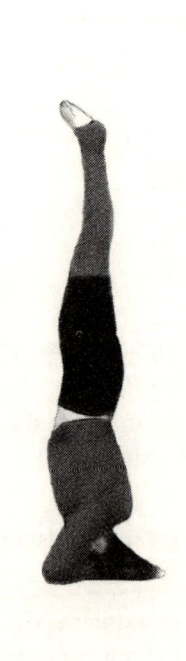

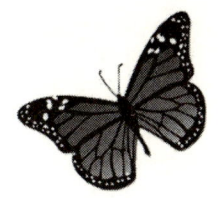

Sutra Five: Trust

Admit to the Divine, to myself, and to another human being, the exact nature of my fears.

In writing our fourth sutra, we begin the process of dissolving the false self. We may feel uncomfortable when we reflect on our behaviors and actions while we were still addicted, But, as we progress through these Sutras, we discern the contours of our story and individualized identity or personality.

As we move into the fifth sutra, we can acknowledge to our Higher Self that we have now made a distinction between the false and the true. We are willing to shed whatever no longer serves our highest good. Awareness begins to blossom.

I recall a story a friend told me about a man who was serving time in prison. My friend was teaching Prison Smart, an Art of Living breathing and meditation course held in prisons. As this man came out of meditation, he began sobbing. He looked at my friend and said, "I'm so sorry. I didn't know." At that moment, this man had the awareness that he was much larger than his mistake. He had gone from ignorance to awareness, which is one function of Sudarshan Kriya Yoga (SKY), yoga, and meditation.

From Denial to Acknowledgment

We are slowly moving out of the tamasic state of inertia and denial. Our true essence is revealed. We see that our actions and behaviors were motivated by desires that are manifestations of the individualized jeeva whose function is to act, accomplish, and attain. The distinction between our self and our Higher Self is more clearly understood, as explained in *Vedanta: The Science of Life*: "The Self is All-pervading, perfect and, as such, there is no desire in it. When desires are no more, actions cannot originate from there. In the Self, there are no desires, and so, the Self neither acts nor gets reacted."[1]

Acknowledgment is the first step in distinguishing between the real and the unreal. When self-acknowledgment arises, the walls of denial begin to crumble. The fifth sutra requires honesty and self-disclosure. This transparency promotes the authenticity and trust that is required for a lasting relationship with our sponsor, ourselves, and, ultimately the Divine.

I remember first entering psychotherapy after a stay in a drug and alcohol detoxification unit. I would find myself lying to my own therapist out of fear of being judged. She once told me, "I cannot help you if you are not honest with me." Because she had been in recovery as well, I eventually developed a trusting bond with her.

We begin by trusting someone who has walked the path before us and who has had similar experiences, but who has also demonstrated consistent effort and commitment to recovery. We seek out a mentor who has found solutions to dealing with life in a better way. The anxiety, fear, and depression that are common when we begin our journey out of the grip of addiction are directly related to thoughts and past impressions, often stemming from trauma, that have been stored in our memory. Dr. Peter Levine, an expert on the topic of trauma, points out, "The paradox of trauma is that it has the power to destroy and the power to transform and resurrect. Whether trauma will be a cruel and punishing Gorgon, or a vehicle for soaring to the heights of transformation and mastery, depends upon how we approach it."[2] When we open up and share these undesirable memories about ourselves and others, we clear away past, stagnant energy. Levine further states, "In being able to harness these primordial and intelligent energies, we can move through trauma and transform it."[3] These memories no longer torture us.

Banishing Resentment and Building Trust

The fifth sutra is a resentment-eviction process. We are freeing ourselves from the bondage of our past, and whatever no longer serves us as we move forward in life. Bringing light to our shadow allows for healing. Building trust diminishes doubt.

In yoga, *sirsasana,* or headstand, is a useful tool to build trust. Much like your life's state of affairs in early recovery, things may be upside down.

Your situation is uncomfortable and alien to you. The ego will place fearful thoughts in your mind, conning you into believing you cannot persevere. But you realize that your life needed to be turned upside down so you could see from a different angle. Now you can build from the bottom up and create a strong foundation. This is the beginner's mind, or "Zen mind."

Doubt is a dark cloud that can block our Divinity and connection to our Source. Doubt generates uncertainty and exacerbates fear. Trusting in the Twelve-Sutra process is essential in early recovery because we have no tangible evidence that our life is improving yet. The fifth sutra creates the space necessary to construct a new life by banishing resentments from the past.

After attending twelve-step meetings for several years, I picked up a phrase that resonated with me: "You cannot be in fear and faith at the same time." Fear and faith are distinctly different qualities of consciousness, meaning if I am experiencing fear, I have shifted away from faith; one state takes over. Marianne Williamson writes, "Faith is an aspect of consciousness. We either have faith in fear or we have faith in love, faith in the power of the world or faith in the power of God."[4] Addicted individuals are innately driven by fear; therefore, it is crucial to build trust and faith to shift our consciousness in that direction.

Establishing trust in someone else is important, but it is only a pathway to developing trust within ourselves. At the beginning of our journey, we need guidance, so we may seek a sponsor who can lead us along the spiritual twelve-step path. Ultimately, the path will lead us to ourselves, or our true Self, where all questions dissolve.

I remember consulting with my sponsor when I was considering a geographical move. I was living in Chicago, but my heart longed to come back to Los Angeles, where I first found recovery. My sponsor asked, "What does your gut say?" She was urging me to follow my inner, higher guidance, which never steers us in the wrong direction. The very fact that I was even contemplating this decision suggests that my Higher Self was attempting to get my attention. When I followed this internal guidance and moved back to LA, many of my intentions manifested, including finishing my graduate degree; seven years later having recovered, I had finally returned to my university and finished my master's program.

After working the fifth sutra, we are delivered from isolation. We have developed a connection with someone and we have laid the groundwork necessary to forge a connection with our Divine Self. All that is false is beginning to fade away as more and more light begins to shine on our truth or Divinity within. We are uncovering, discovering, and discarding. We are free of secrets that keep us imprisoned in a state of anxiety and fear. We are liberated from the bondage of the false self. Our doubts dissolve as trust emerges. We realize that the instances in which we doubt ourselves become the exact opportunities we need to build trust in ourselves and in our Higher Power, or God.

After several years of continuing to relapse, I doubted my ability to achieve one year clean and sober. But I had the tools of the twelve sutras and faith and in my guru, Sri Sri Ravi Shankar. I knew that his grace and guidance would see me through any difficulty. When doubt arose in my mind, I would extinguish it with my faith. Soon, days became weeks, and weeks became months, and I eventually made it to one year clean and sober.

When we discard remnants of fear and darkness that taint the purity of our essence, we illuminate our soul. We become conscious of the darkness. This consciousness is the wick from which the flame shines more brightly. The consciousness that emerges allows us to be free and liberate ourselves from our past. As Swami Chinmayananda notes:

"Even to say there is darkness, we must be conscious of it. The 'Light' of awareness is so subtle and Absolute, that it illumines not only the various sources of light in the world, but also the experience of darkness itself. That which illumines both light and darkness must be a factor that transcends both these experiences. Therefore, the Spirit is indicated as that which transcends the darkness."[5]

The greatest gift we receive from working the twelve sutras is awareness, or the ability to see ourselves clearly. We create an objective lens through which we are able to magnify our image. The further we move forward working the sutras, the more clearly we see that the "darkness" is not who we are but an accumulation of actions and behaviors carried out in ignorance or lack of awareness.

Why a Sponsor?

We share our past with another person because we need the safety to express ourselves free of judgment. It is also imperative to disclose our mistakes in the fifth sutra so that our sponsor can provide an objective eye and make us aware of our defects or repetitive patterns that have kept us in the cycle of active addiction. These defects will eventually need to be replaced with spiritual principles if we want to live with the Higher-Mind and create a solid foundation that will enable us to live a healthy, peaceful, productive life.

Trust is complete reliance that the universe is guiding us at all times. We all experience synchronicities or "divine" coincidences that occur throughout our lives. But if we pay attention, these occurrences are happening every moment in each and every human encounter. A Higher Power communicates through us and among us all day. We simply need to be open to receive the spiritual cues. We are literally being guided and supported 24/7, but we must be receptive to this guidance and support.

For example, as I was writing this chapter and thinking through the virtue of trust, I had a divine encounter. I decided to take a break from writing, so I stepped outside my apartment complex to get some fresh air. I walked to the fountain and sat on a bench. Nearby, on the opposite bench, a girl was sitting by herself. I felt guided to reach out to her, so I approached her and sat beside her. I greeted her warmly and asked her name. She told me her name was Shraddha. *Shraddha* in Sanskrit means "trust" or "faith." After conversing with her, I also found out that we were connected to the same guru, Sri Sri Ravi Shankar. At once, I had an aha moment.

How was it that I had chosen that exact moment during the day to take a break?

Every moment becomes an unspoken encounter with the Divine. The key is to continue to stay connected to the Source. Through consistent spiritual practice, we clear our channel so that we stay tuned in. When we develop this sense of trust, we become comfortable with the unknown, even excited about the possibilities the unknown presents. When we trust, we let go of fear and embrace life with ease.

Trust that you are being given exactly what you need at this moment and that your dharma is being revealed to you in each situation. Trust in the Higher Consciousness as a road map to your highest evolution.

Now, It's Your Turn:

1) Think of one situation in your life now where doubt exists. It could be related to a person, place, or situation.
2) Now, what action would you need to take to turn that doubt into trust?
3) Do you need to have an important conversation with someone?
4) Do you need to ask for guidance, or simply pray about it?

C'mon. S-T-R-E-T-C-H! You're building something extraordinary, it's worth it!

In Sutra Three, we aligned our will with a Power greater than our small self, or our finite self. Now trust in that Power as your internal navigation system. Embrace your daily divine encounters because they are guideposts along your journey. Open up to the Power that surrounds you and be grateful that surrendering has allowed you to stretch beyond, into a realm where the ultimate power of manifestation and co-creation dwells.

In Hindu culture, the goddess Parvati is known as the goddess of power, creation, and victory over good and evil. Parvati is the source of all powers and weapons and she is used as the base for doing any work. Parvati is Shiva's wife in ancient Indian mythology. She is known as the Daughter of the Mountain. Parvati and Shiva's relationship represent the balance between renunciation and worldly pursuits. In a healthy partnership, resides trust. Trust in Divinity breeds trust in one's life. In Sutra Five, we trust that a Power greater than our finite self is leading us to our destiny.

SUTRA SIX

DEITY: Kali

PRINCIPLE: Fortitude

MANTRA: *Om Devi Namo Namah*
(I bow to the goddess of courage, strength, and power)

ASANA: *Rajakapotasana* (king pigeon pose)

MEDITATION: Find a quiet spot to sit for five minutes with your eyes closed and repeat ten times:

"Bestow on me the ability to see, through the storm, I transform."

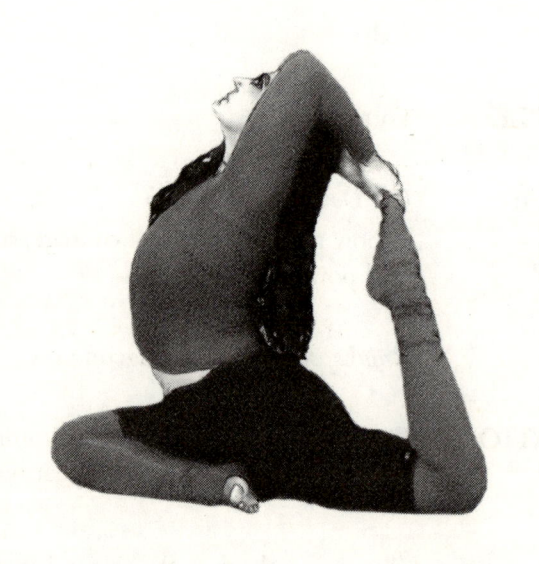

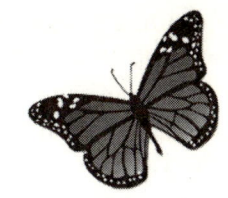

Sutra Six: Fortitude

Become entirely ready to have the Divine restore me to Love

In Sutra Five, we admitted to God, to ourselves, and to another human being the exact nature of our wrongs. As we move on to Sutra Six, we will uncover the nature of our wrongs. We get a clear understanding of our character defects, or those qualities that keep us stuck in repetitive patterns of behavior that no longer promote our spiritual advancement.

When we truly look at the root or nature of our wrongs, we see that our defects all stem from fear. We see the fearful illusions projected outward through the ego's identification with the material realm or the need to satisfy the small self.

For example, after working my fifth sutra, the central character defect that was brought to my attention was impatience. Impatience was a common theme in my life. I had to examine the driving force behind this impatience. In all my attempts at recovery, I would consistently make it to nine months clean/sober and then relapse. The repetitive pattern was that I would get nine months sober, think I was fully recovered, and then leave my sober living or recovery home. I would venture out into the world for FOMO (Fear Of Missing Out). A strong foundation was never fully constructed, so the house would always crumble to the ground. I was afraid that I was running out of time to establish myself in the world.

Once I understood how my fear manifested as impatience, I was able to act differently—not according to fear but according to the universe's plan, which has its own timeline. I accepted that all things occur on the divine clock, not my watch, and I cultivated the virtue of patience. In doing so, I was able to build a solid foundation in recovery that afforded me the opportunity to achieve my worldly goals.

In Vedantic philosophy, there are six types of emotions that arise in the ignorant mind: *kama* (desire), *krodha* (anger), *lobha* (greed), *moha* (delusion), *mada* (passion), and *matsarya* (jealousy).[1] These character deficits are attached to rajas (activity) and maya (illusion), and cause agitation in the mind. When we desire something and we do not possess the means to obtain it, anger or frustration may arise. Swami Chidbhavananda writes:

"Mind gets disturbed and depraved every time desire, fear and anger make their evil appearance in it. The reflection of an object gets hazy and broken on the surface of disturbed water. Likewise the presence of Atman is obscured in a disturbed mind. It should first of all gain quietude through the conquest of desire, fear and anger. Meditation then becomes easy and spontaneous."[2]

Indeed, when we seek pleasure or gratification from the unreal, or from an object in maya, we will never truly feel content because objects can never bring sustained contentment. Overcoming these aspects of rajas through nonattachment alleviates suffering.

The Root of an Addicted Individual's Suffering

In active addiction, there is an inherent need to fulfill the small self. This self-centered structure, known as *asmita*, is the root of an addict's suffering. Desire, or the craving to acquire something to bolster our sense of self, perpetuates suffering. When a part of the egoic structure, asmita, becomes afraid of losing something or experiences a diminished identity, it lashes out. Matsarya (jealousy) is an example of this phenomenon. Jealousy originates from fear. We are afraid of losing something so we compensate by being overprotective, possessive, or manipulative. These are all character defects. Jealousy stems from a mindset of lack, but we must remember that what is ours will always be ours; it won't pass us by. An attitudinal deficit can be countered by an attitude of abundance and by knowing that we have everything we need at this moment. According to the *Big Book of Alcoholics Anonymous*, "Driven by a hundred forms of fear, self-delusion, self-seeking, and self-pity, we step on the toes of others and they retaliate."[3] In the *Bhagavad Gita*, there is a verse that illustrates this process in the mind:

"Brooding on the objects of senses, man develops attachment to them; from attachment comes desire; from desire anger sprouts. From anger proceeds delusion; from delusion, confused memory; from confused memory the ruin of reason; due to the ruin of reason, he perishes."[4]

In active addiction, our character defects prompt unreasonable behavior, such as lying, manipulating, stealing, and acts of violence. This kind of behavior inevitably makes life insane and chaotic.

Learn to become the observer of your own mind. When you notice fear arising or you observe the fear-factor movie playing out in your mind, simply refrain from clinging to those thoughts and the fear will dissipate. Observe your own thoughts through detached awareness. When you believe these fearful thoughts to be true, you will have a coinciding experience and react from this place. For example, I struggled with seeking certainty by calling psychics. My mind would get stuck in fear and worry and I would have the urge to speak to a psychic in order to gain clarity, however, my behavior was fear-driven; an unhealthy reaction to a fleeting thought. In time, I learned to surrender the need for certainty and rely on my Higher Power, thus, not acting out the behavior. My character defect arose from fear and could only be countered by cultivating trust.

In my early days of recovery, I was afraid that I would relapse. My thoughts were always centered around a struggle. I was told that I had a fatal illness—addiction—that was incurable and that I would suffer for the rest of my life. Because I was so fearful that I would relapse, all I could think about was preventing a relapse. As a result, I would continue to relapse. Where your attention goes, energy flows. This was when I decided to shift my focus to being fully recovered.

What you resist persists. What you focus on takes up residence in your mind and your life. Until I reprogrammed my mind to think kind, loving thoughts, such as "I'm whole, perfect, and complete" and "I am restored to perfect health," I was not able to achieve long-term sobriety. This is the magnitude of the power of thought.

Another form of suffering is known as avidya, or ignorance. When we identify what is unreal with the real or the non-atman with the atman, we become attached to maya. If we identify with the ego, we get lost in the egoic illusion. If I believe that a person, place, or thing will make me happy, then I fall into this trap.

Objects in maya seem seductive. They are alluring but thinking that we become whole from objects in the material realm is ignorance. This ignorance stems from delusions in the mind. The mind is the source of our ignorance and our suffering. Hence, working the twelve sutras is a method of unlearning ignorance and recognizing truth.

In *Vedanta: The Science of Life*, Swami Chinmayanada states:

"Apart from the mind there is no ignorance (Avidya). The mind itself is the ignorance which is the cause for the bondage of rebirth. When the mind is destroyed, everything else is destroyed. When the mind manifests, everything else manifests. All Avidya put together is Maya. Therefore other than the mind, there is no Avidya. Mind alone is Avidya. It is the cause for all the bondages."[5]

The way to reestablish awareness or equanimity in the mind and to overcome avidya is to acquire knowledge. When the mind becomes saturated with truth, there is no room for ignorance. Once we confront our character defects, we cannot revert back to a state of ignorance. If we do regress, we can always return to knowledge.

Knowledge provides awareness and awareness points us in the direction of the truth. Knowledge prompts us to understand the distinction between the real, atman and Brahman, and the nonreal, maya. Knowledge provides us with the framework to discover who we really are, which is the not the identity reflected in our character defects. Our essence is love, joy, and peace. The Bhagavad Gita beautifully illustrates this point:

"Shining like the sun, knowledge reveals the Supreme in them, in whom ignorance is destroyed by Self-knowledge. Darkness vanishes when the sun rises; ignorance dies with the dawn of knowledge. As sunlight reveals form and gives life, Self-knowledge or Brahma-jnanam poses the Reality of Brahman and the evanescence of Prakriti. The knower of Brahman knows he is Brahman and none else"[6]

The Virtue of Fortitude

Being *entirely ready* suggests a heightened level of willingness—willingness to let go of whatever clouds our essence and keeps us in a cycle of destructive behavior. We must be willing to let go of whatever seems familiar and secure and replace that with something much more life-sustaining. Our willingness leads to fortitude, or endurance in times of adversity, which transforms our moral landscape.

In Hindu mythology, Kali is the dark goddess of power and destruction. Kali puts an end to illusion. Known as the Dark One, Kali has a somewhat demonic and frightening appearance. She is the feminine manifestation of Shiva, the destroyer; the dark slayer of demonic forces. She is depicted wearing slaughtered heads, symbolizing the destruction of the mind. We must slay our mental vices or character defects to progress on the spiritual path. Darkness cannot exist without light and vice versa. The word Kali also relates to Kaal or time. Time eats all. The heads that Kali wears is a reminder that all that is born will die. The inevitability of death brings us back to the value of life.

Again, opposite values are complementary. Facing adversity, moving through it, and making it to the other side, is a natural part of recovery and healing. Essentially, this sutra cannot be skipped, as it takes looking squarely at our shadow side and making necessary changes. This resoluteness is key in overcoming life's battles. As the saying goes, "Nothing changes, if nothing changes."

It has been my experience working this Sutra that when I become willing, I am presented with more opportunities that allow me to recognize and overcome my character defects and fear-based patterns. One of my most prominent character defects, impatience, continually came up as I was working this Sutra. In order to overcome this defect, the universe repeatedly put situations in my path that required me to consciously scrutinize my impatience.

I would be driving and run into traffic everywhere I went. Practicing fortitude by patiently enduring the traffic jam stops my normal impulsive reaction to become frustrated and honk at the person in front of me. Acknowledging the defect as it arises gives us the awareness not to act on it, but instead, to allow it to pass.

In yoga, the posture *eka pada rajakapotasana,* or one-legged king pigeon pose, is a deep hip opener. The hips are huge emotional storage depots. Sitting in this posture is sometimes painful and uncomfortable, but when we endure the pain, we release it. In order to move beyond the pain, we must move through it. Nothing is permanent. Pain and happiness are fleeting emotions and will always pass. By withstanding the discomfort, we cultivate patience and allow things to subside.

Impatience in the mind creates uneasiness. A character defect is overcome by practicing the opposite. The guru Sri Sri Ravi Shankar's principle is this: "Patience in the mind, and dynamism in action."

Now, It's Your Turn:

1) First, make a list of your character defects on the left, next list their opposite assets on the right.
2) Now, identify instances in which each character defect arises
3) What is one action you can take when the defect surfaces that would increase the character asset (opposite of defect)?

<u>Character Defects (list them)</u>   <u>Character Assets (list them)</u>

Here's my example:
Character Defect: Impatience   **Character Asset:** Patience
Instances in which defect arises: Driving in traffic, not hearing back from someone
Action: Pray (action) and ask the Divine to help me be patient and trust in the unfolding of life

Now it's your turn. How can you gain awareness and combat character defects?

Character Defect: **Character Asset:**
Instances in which it arises:
Action:

Paradoxically, we are far more dynamic and effective when we act from a still, patient mind. The sixth sutra allows us to change the entire paradigm of our lives by recognizing our defects and making subtle shifts in the opposing direction.

For example, if I am judging someone, I am judgmental. Recognizing that this defect exists within the egoic structure of my mind gives me the opportunity to change my state of consciousness to one of acceptance. The recognition, or awareness, of this defect is the space that causes the defect to dissipate, dissolve, or shift into its opposite character asset.

Sutra Six provides us with the awareness necessary to see a distinct separation between "I," the false self, and the divine Self, which is formless and infinite. In the Vedas, this is separation between the jeeva (ego) and the atman (soul), or illusion and reality.

In Brahman, we are connected to everything and everyone in this universe. It is only the individualized ego, or jeeva, that places any value on separation. So our defects spring from the ego's function of separation or individualism. When we further establish our connection to Divinity or the Source, the need for separation dissipates and the ego's primacy diminishes.

The Role of Meditation

One valuable tool that allows us to maintain our connection to the Source and develop this detached awareness is meditation. Pacifying mental activity and reposing in a state of *samadhi* (intense absorption) keeps us connected to our truth. The more we experience our truth, the more divinely aligned our actions become. Swami Chinmayananda elaborates:

"The more one attunes one's mind to the truth, the more one gains equilibrium. The truth is, the Lord is the invisible propeller of all actions in the universe. He is the true owner of everything sentient and insentient. Man's prerogative is to know this truth and to adjust his life activities accordingly. His mental fever gets pacified in that way. Further efficiency in the execution of duty increases in him."[7]

SUTRA SEVEN

DEITY: Ganesha

PRINCIPLE: Humility

MANTRA: *Om Namo Ganeshaya*
(I pray to the remover of obstacles)

ASANA: *Uttanasana* (standing forward bend)

MEDITATION: Find a quiet spot and sit comfortably with your eyes closed. Repeat ten times:

"Brought to my knees, I am humble and free."

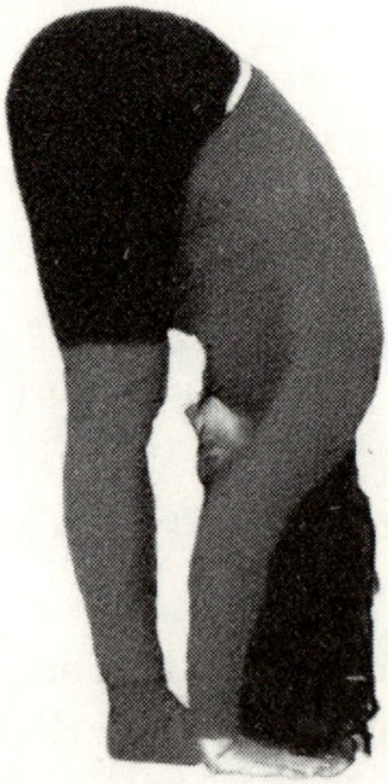

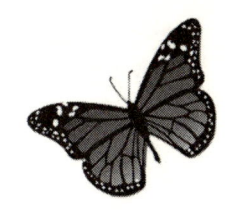

Sutra Seven: Humility

*Humbly ask the Divine
to instill Love where there is fear*

The fundamental principle of Sutra Seven is humility. This step requires a new level of honesty. We honestly assess our intentions and motives. We carefully monitor our actions, making sure that we are not acting out of defects that were revealed in Sutra Six. Now that we are aware that these defects exist and have caused much of our suffering and the progression of the addiction, we have a responsibility to alter our actions. Each of our shortcomings is an action born from a defect.

For example, I may be experiencing anger, or there may be anger present in my mind, but if I decide to yell at someone, projecting my anger outward, I have just reacted or displayed a shortcoming. That is, a shortcoming arises when a negative thought is translated into action. Recognize that your thoughts will allow you to observe the mind without dictating an action. You are the co-creator of your life and if you want to create harmony in your external world, then you must learn to be in sync with your essence and to act in accordance with love.

Humility has a distinct function. The aspect of our existence that chooses to act or react from a place of fear will struggle to survive and guide our actions if we are not continually humbled. Through humility, we place our feet more firmly on the spiritual path and become more aware of who we really are. We realign our behaviors and actions with our true nature, our divine Self.

Humility deflates the ego. It is the compass that guides us home. Without some level of suffering, humility cannot be understood and experienced. This is why it is sometimes necessary for addicted individuals to "hit a bottom." Hitting a bottom literally thrusts the ego to the floor, allowing rebirth and transformation to occur. Humility forces us to see that ultimately we have no control. Humility is being honest about our circumstances, our part in creating them, and who we really are.

The Synergy of Renunciation and Action

Sutra Seven incorporates both renunciation, nivritti, and action, pravritti. We renounce whatever no longer serves us and we take action to recognize our defects, gain awareness not to act upon them, eliminate our shortcomings (fear-driven behaviors), and strengthen our roots in love.

Sutras One to Three are nivritti steps–renunciation and preparation for progress. Sutras Four to Nine are pravritti steps because they require action, and action is the vehicle for tangible progress and results. Then in Sutras Ten to Twelve, we return to nivritti. Both renunciation and action are equally important because we cannot have stability without progress or progress without stability. Again, opposite values are complementary.

For example, my ability to write (action–pravritti) strongly relies on my spiritual practices (renunciation–nivritti). Without conscious contact with the Divine Source, creativity cannot flow easily; creativity is a by-product of meditation. Life is an interdependent system.

Character defects spring from fear. Humility prevents fearful thoughts from manifesting into fearful actions. I consciously strive to keep my ego in check and this allows me to truly be myself and not act out of fear, which is where defects originate.

Being humble keeps our actions aligned with love and therefore raises our vibration level. The closer we are to love, the higher our vibration because love is the universal frequency. It's naturally where the universe wants us to dwell. When we act from a place of love, we uplift those around us. Humility suppresses the ego and aligns us with Higher-Consciousness. Spiritual practices allow us to connect to ourselves and reaffirm our true nature, which is love. It is not possible to intellectually exude love. Intellectually we can distinguish between fear and love, or between the atman (Self) and the jeeva (ego), but we must experience the Divinity within in order to cultivate that presence and live from that space.

The principle of humility is exemplified by the Hindu god Ganesha. Ganesha is the remover of obstacles. If you see a statue or picture of Ganesha, there is a small mouse under his feet. This mouse represents the ego in relation to the greater universal Divinity. Half man, half elephant, Ganesha represents the macrocosm and microcosm. The elephant is the human potential for enlightenment. Some people seek Divine help and guidance only in times of turmoil because there is a level of desperation and human devices have failed. In the wake of destruction and darkness, it is the humbling of one's spirit that moves mountains, symbolic of Ganesha's power to remove obstacles, allowing access to enlightenment and success. When the ego is set aside, humility allows one to start over in a surrendered state.

In yoga, *uttanasana* (standing forward bend) is a posture in which we fold forward from the hips, letting the head hang down toward the feet. This symbolizes reverence and humility. In China, it is a custom to bow in reverence, acknowledging our elders and superiors. We recognize our inferior nature in the grand scheme.

The ego has its place and when it humbly sits beneath the Divine, it does not get in the way of the divine light shining forth. Ego is a barrier to spiritual development if we choose to act according to its wishes and demands. The ego embodies a sense of entitlement, separation, and uniqueness, all qualities that prevent us from experiencing the ultimate interconnectedness of all. There is a divine bond between all humans.

In *Ransoming the Mind,* international lecturer, yogi, and meditation expert Yogiraj Charles Bates writes of the ego:

"It is the ego in the void, that which is void of attachment to separateness crying, "It is I." The I-ness seeks to maintain its self-existence and to do so, must ignore the reality of "there is only one" or "there is truly none." It must maintain its separateness in order to achieve and preserve its sense of identity. It asserts and maintains this by viewing things other than itself."[1]

Suffering stems from the ego's affinity to satisfy itself. When we place our wants and needs above fulfilling our dharma, something will inevitably happen to rein in our ego. Throughout our active addiction, identification with ego repeatedly brought us to our knees. Our bottoms progressively became lower and lower. We were forced into a state of humility through repeated humiliation.

Receiving a DUI and spending time in jail were humbling experiences for me. It was humiliating for me to stand in a courtroom wearing an orange jumpsuit with my feet shackled, as I witnessed my mother with tears streaming down her face. In the *Twelve Steps and Twelve Traditions*, Step 7 makes the following point, "It was only at the end of a long road, marked by successive defeats and humiliations, and the final crushing of our self-sufficiency, that we began to feel humility as something more than a condition of groveling despair."[2]

Now, It's Your Turn:

Ego Deflation:
1) List one or more instances in your life when you felt humiliated.
2) How did the event humble you?
3) How did it make you stronger and wiser?
4) Be grateful for those events because they are eye-openers to your truth.

5) Now make a gratitude list and name ten people, places, things, events, or situations that have helped you on your spiritual path.

The virtue of humility reminds me of words of wisdom I learned from a respected teacher and friend. She told me, "Walk like a queen without ego." It almost seems counterintuitive, but "my" achievements and assets are not really "mine." In *Freedom from Addiction*, Deepak Chopra writes, "Likewise before awakening, the ego takes credit for its accomplishments, but upon recognizing its true nature becomes lightheartedly humble."[3]

I am not the doer. The more I recognize and align myself with this fundamental concept, the easier and more fluid my life becomes. The small self, asmita, or the mouse beneath Ganesha's foot, is only as influential as I allow it to be.

When we rely on our higher consciousness to propel us forward, we do not encounter external resistance. Humbly affirming our limited mortal capabilities keeps our feet firmly planted on spiritual soil, which becomes fertile ground for pure possibility and divine manifestation.

SUTRA EIGHT

DEITY: Hanuman

PRINCIPLE: Forgiveness

MANTRA: *Jai Bajrang Bali Hanuman* (Victory to Lord Hanuman).

(Chanted as a prayer for strength before commencing anything that requires hard work or is challenging)

ASANA: *Hanumanasana* (full splits)

MEDITATION: Find a quiet spot to sit for at least five minutes. Close your eyes and repeat ten times:

"Through forgiveness I forge ahead, my destiny's tracks I tread."

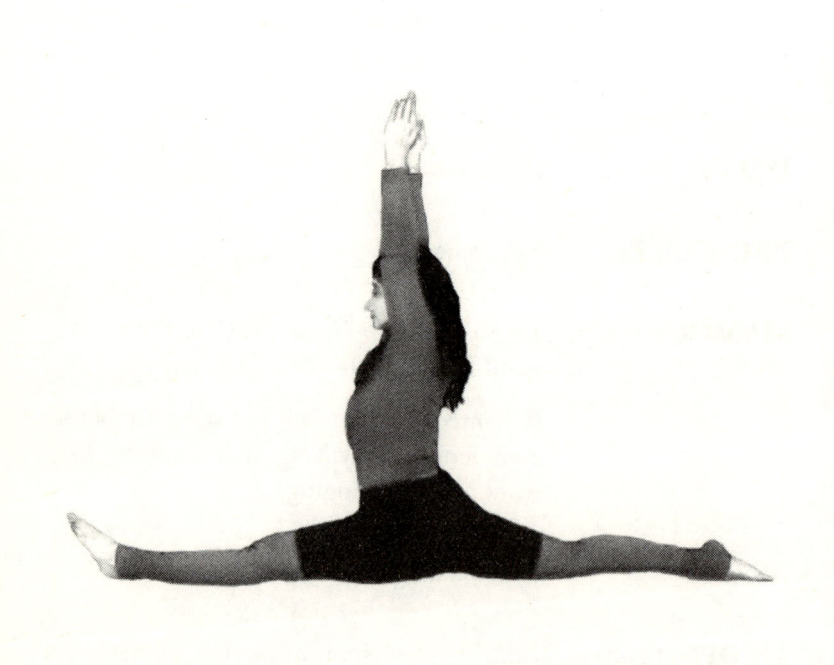

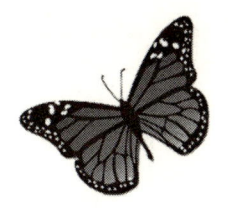

Sutra Eight: Forgiveness

Make a list of all persons I may have harmed and become willing to restore Love

In Sutra Eight, we recognize that we must scrutinize the karma we have created throughout our addiction and assess how our actions have affected our relationships. In the *Twelve Steps and Twelve Traditions*, Step Eight states:

"First we take a look backward and try to discover where we have been at fault; next we make a vigorous attempt to repair the damage we have done; and third, having thus cleaned away the debris of the past, we consider how, with our newfound knowledge of ourselves, we may develop the best possible relations with every human being we know."[1]

We begin to size up our accumulated karma, preparing for Sutra Nine where we will clear out our karma. Fear and anxiety may develop as we confront our karmic history. However, hopefully, making the list and making an honest appraisal of the harm we have caused others will prevent us from creating more wreckage. Moving forward, we seek to take conscious action. We begin to apply the yoga of action, or karma yoga, to our lives.

This sutra is crucial because it is our duty, or dharma, to amend our acts of ignorance. We must take responsibility for where and how we may have inflicted spiritual harm. We begin to take "god-ward" action, or actions that move us toward higher spiritual evolution. As awareness develops and ignorance fades, we arrive at what the *Big Book of Alcoholics Anonymous* calls the "fourth dimension," or a higher spiritual plane.

Swami Vivekananda explains, "Any action that makes us go Godward is a good action and is our duty."[2] This is the underlying theme of karma yoga.

Universal law pushes us toward spiritual evolution. We must continue to progress on that path. Failure to recognize our dharma, take responsibility, and pursue conscious action only creates stagnation. Eventually, some divinely orchestrated event will force us to expand, transform, and move in the direction that is most harmonious to the universe.

The greatest story of duty is that of Arjuna in the Bhagavad Gita. Arjuna must go into battle with his own cousins, but he hesitates to do so. He understands the ramifications fighting his own kin will create. He does not wish to engage in such a battle, but Lord Krishna urges him to take up arms because it is dharma; righteous duty as a warrior.

The Bhagavad Gita notes, "With these perplexing words, you are, as it were, confusing my comprehension. Tell me with certainty the path by pursuing which I may get at the Supreme"(Chapter III, verse 2). Commenting on this, Swami Chidbhavananda explains, "The lord made it plain to Arjuna that he was not to abandon his duty for any reason whatsoever. After goading him to action, he instructed Arjuna to convert the bondage-creating karma into bondage-breaking karma."[3]

Settling Karmic Debts

Our addiction has been our bondage and we are liberated from this bondage by settling our karmic debts. We must make positive karmic deposits into our spiritual bank account. We must build good karmic credit to be made trustworthy again. We need to atone for our negative actions that may have caused others suffering or pain. However, it is important to be aware that we are not trying to persecute ourselves for our past karma. After all, we acted out of ignorance; if we had been aware of the implications of our actions, our choices most likely would have been different.

An intoxicated, tamasic mind will invariably act from a state of ignorance, influencing us to make poor choices that yield poor results. A rajasic mind, riddled with craving, creates thoughts based on attachment to worldly, mundane objects or desires.

When our desire for something is greater than our compassion for the person who may suffer as a result of our fulfilling that desire, we inflict pain on ourselves and others, and rack up karmic debt. But if we maintain a sattvic pure state of mind, in which contentment, peace, and love guide our actions, our actions will produce spiritually sustaining karma. From such a level of consciousness, we gain true liberation from the bondage of ego.

My desire for intoxicants was stronger than my compassion and consideration for my family. I later discovered that I could achieve the same effect—a euphoric state of bliss—from Sudarshan Kriya, yoga, and meditation. In *Overcoming Addictions*, Deepak Chopra describes addicted individuals as "misguided seekers"[4] looking for a solution that can only be found within. Chopra goes on to discuss the need for spiritual fulfillment and the chase for *ecstasy*. We humans can forget the true source of this bliss, winding up lost on a never-ending search.

Many addicted individuals are simply not able to recover because they continue to chase the initial high they felt when they first experienced the drug-induced effects. The memory of the high is associated with the drug. Until they replace the drug with a natural, life-sustaining, spiritual substitute, the futile search will continue. But for that, samskaras must be wiped clean and past karma burned.

So what exactly is an amend? An amend is reparation for harm we impose on others and ourselves. We must make amends to ourselves and this can only happen through forgiveness. Forgiveness allows us to rewrite our story, freeing us from the bondage of our past. *A Course in Miracles* states, "For forgiveness literally transforms vision, and lets you see the real world reaching quietly and gently across chaos, removing all illusions that had twisted your perception and fixed it on the past."[5]

Donning Spiritual Armor

The moment we forgive, we are free. But we must be willing to let go of everything that we think is true about ourselves. Our actions and behaviors in the past were a projection of ego-driven chaos. So, we must truly be ready to step out of chaos and self-defeating patterns and put our spiritual armor on.

I had an interesting experience while working Step 9 with my sponsor while in a 12-Step fellowship. She had assigned questions for me to answer and asked me to define a few words. I am a work-driven person, with an "A-student" perfectionist personality, so I took the assignment seriously and made the time to fully work through the step. When we sat down to review my work, I suddenly realized that I had completely overlooked one question: "What is forgiveness?" To my surprise, I had unconsciously skipped this question, even though I thought I had thoroughly completed the step. We both laughed because, obviously, God was directing me to spend more time contemplating the meaning of forgiveness. When I returned home and continued my writing, I realized that I had not fully forgiven myself or others for the past. I was not ready to move forward until I became willing to forgive. I have a choice—I can either condemn or I can forgive. The latter always leads to freedom.

At age thirty-three, I successfully managed to get clean from opiates and prescription pills, but I was still being prescribed antidepressants. In the opinion of my parents (both physicians), this was the best treatment for my depression. After being on "legally prescribed drugs" for the majority of my life, my entire physical, mental, and emotional chemistry had changed. The antidepressants were becoming as harmful, if not more harmful, than the opiates.

I decided to become medication/drug-free. I practiced a breathing technique called Sudarshan Kriya Yoga (SKY), taught by the Art of Living Foundation, for three months consistently and my body began to expel the toxins in the medication. I followed my intuition, which was becoming increasingly sharp, and weaned myself off all medication, against my psychiatrist's recommendation. I was ecstatic at the positive impact this had on me. Once I was completely chemical-free, I felt like myself again. My creativity bloomed and my cognitive functions improved.

Even though I was grateful to finally feel "normal," I harbored a deep resentment against my parents. I felt as if I had been robbed of years of my adult life. I did not understand how they could choose to medicate me, rather than search for alternative, healthy methods of treatment.

After deep introspection, I realized that people who care about us help the best way they know how. If they had known the long-term effects psychotropic medication had on me, my parents may have chosen an alternative path for me. The anger and resentment I directed toward my parents in the past was causing me pain in the present. I extend compassion toward them now because their actions came from a place of love and concern. Their intentions were honorable.

The challenges I faced from the addictive effects of medication became the springboard I needed to help others. The crisis became the opportunity. It has been my repeated experience that the Divine will "bring you to it and pull you through it." I had to forgive and let go in order to move forward.

In the Indian epic, *Ramayana,* the god Hanuman helps Rama defeat the evil king Ravana. Hanuman was Rama's companion and devoted sidekick and was known to have possessed great strength. He could perform superhuman tasks, lifting hills and throwing them like stones. There is a famous adage, "Those who live in glass houses should not throw stones," suggesting that those who are vulnerable should not attack others. Forgiveness is taking the higher road and acting from Higher Consciousness. Forgiveness often begins with letting go of guilt and grievances. What distinguished Hanuman from other gods was that he attained divine status simply through his devotion to Rama. In the yogic tradition, this is known as Bhakti yoga. Connection to Divinity is a road to forgiveness, for the Divine is pure love, and is ultimately your true essence.

Recitation of the Hanuman Chalisa prayer invokes Hanuman's divine intervention in grave problems. After receiving a felony DUI, I was arrested and put in jail. I was looking at severe consequences, including lengthy prison time. I found out from my aunt that the night before my hearing, my mother called her to get the Hanuman Chalisa prayer so she could recite it. The next day in court, I was released on my own recognizance. I'm not sure if the Hanuman Chalisa prayer was what helped my situation, but this story did make me realize the importance of forgiveness and appreciating people for their positive qualities. I was able to see my mother in a different light after this and truly forgive. Krishna Das, a beautiful musician and student of Ram Dass, released a compilation (CDs and book) of the Hanuman Chalisa. In it, he shares 40 lyrical verses that give praise to Hanuman.

Free yourself from the past and you will free yourself of anger, guilt, shame, and resentment. These emotions diminish the spirit. There is a beautiful Art of Living teaching on forgiveness. Try this exercise:

Close your eyes and think about a person you cannot forgive. Make a note of how you feel and the sensations in your body. Open your eyes and write down the feelings or sensations. Now think of a person who you totally accept, someone in your life who is easy to accept. Note the sensations and feelings that arise. Again open your eyes and write down how you feel.

Often you will find that bringing to mind people you do not accept or forgive creates a constriction inside of you. No matter the effect on the other person, non-acceptance is troubling your own mind! Hence the AOL point: "Accept situations and people as they are." Doing so, benefits you, saves your own mind.

Now, It's Your Turn:

Who have you harmed as a result of your addiction?
1) List every one of them and the harm you believed you inflicted. Be specific.
2) Do not allow your mind to jump ahead to actually making your amends. The making of amends is the goal of Sutra Nine and we are not there yet. Stay present!

3) Do not fall prey to the ego's trap of persecution—your actions do not define you. Your true essence is being revealed to you—sometimes quickly, sometimes slowly.
4) Now define the word *Forgive*
5) Finally, answer the following question: Am I now willing to forgive myself and others, 100 percent? Be honest. What are you holding on to? *Let it Go!*

In our active addiction, we cling to fear, guilt, and judgment. They are familiar to the ego and we falsely identify with the ego. But the ego's projection of fear is an illusion; it does not really exist. Similarly, our past no longer exists, so to identify with our past is to cling to the unreal. The truth of who we really are can only be experienced in the present moment. *A Course in Miracles* states, "The past becomes the justification for entering into a continuing, unholy alliance with the ego against the present. For the present is forgiveness."[6]

We can choose truth or we can choose the illusion of what was. Even speaking of the past, or reliving your past, keeps the energy alive. Why would you want to keep stale energy alive? It does not serve you. If a negative thought comes to mind, acknowledge it as such and move the energy away from *akasha*. Akasha is the space element and the very first element in creation. It is the ether from which all matter is formed. Matter is nothing more than energy and words are also energy. The words we speak and the thoughts we think create karma. Speak words of truth, wisdom, and love, and that will become your reality.

Have you noticed that people who complain a lot become fixated in a negative reality? It is uncomfortable to be in the presence of negativity because negativity is viral. Thought, speech, action, and deed all contribute to your karma. Glance back at events in your life. Notice when you were happy and upbeat. Were you surrounded by positive people who made your spirit soar? Manifest your thoughts wisely and diligently take karmic inventory in the present moment.

Hanuman faces a huge challenge when he is assigned the task of helping Rama save Sita and defeat Ravana. He becomes fearful when he sees a huge ocean that he must cross; nevertheless, he continues his quest. In *Ramayana for Children*, V. Ramanathan details Hanuman's response: "For the sake of Rama I will do anything. Crossing the ocean is no problem."[7] Hanuman is willing to do anything to serve Rama, an incarnate of God. In yoga, *hanumanasana*, or full splits, symbolizes this giant leap forward. Let go of your past, forgive, and move forward toward the love and abundance that awaits you.

SUTRA NINE

DEITY: Durga

PRINCIPLE: Responsibility

MANTRA: *Om Devi Durgayai Namah* (Salutations to the goddess)

ASANA: *Virabhadrasana* II (warrior II)

MEDITATION: Find a quiet spot to sit with your eyes closed for five minutes. Repeat silently ten times:

"I own and atone; this path leads me home."

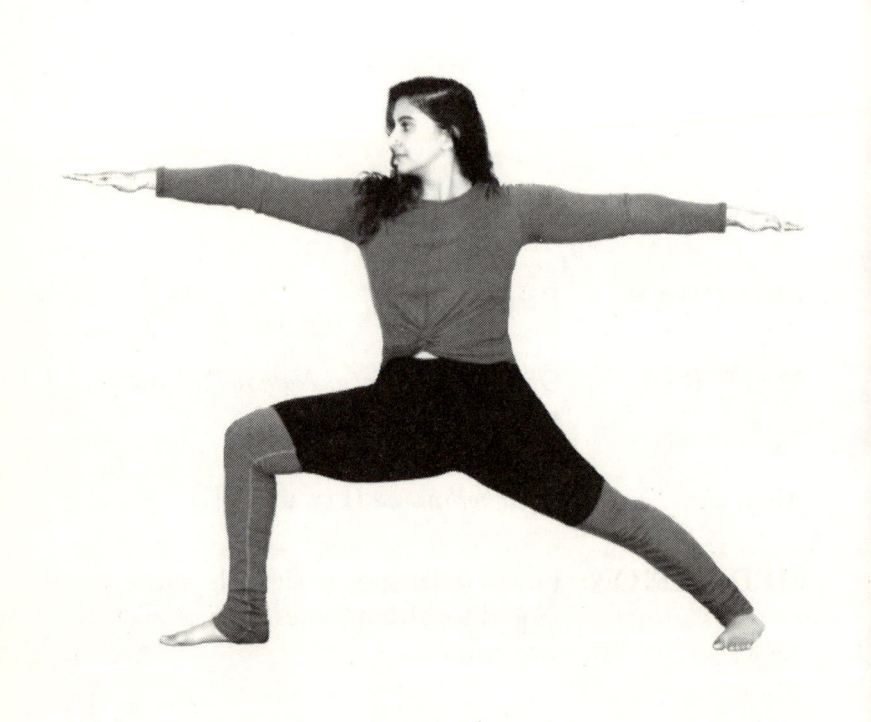

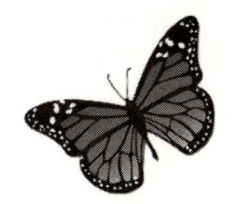

Sutra Nine: Responsibility

Make direct amends to such people wherever possible, with careful and thoughtful consideration for the other.

Sutra Nine is about taking responsibility and then taking action. We were willing to make our list of the people we have harmed in Sutra Eight; now we must become even more willing to follow through with the Twelve-Sutra process. A heightened level of motivation and action is crucial for this sutra.

The ego may instinctively marshal resistance to making direct amends, coming up with rationalizations as to why it may not be necessary to humble ourselves and face people we may have caused spiritual and/or emotional harm. But despite this resistance we must propel ourselves into action. This is the last of the cleansing and release sutras, and the Twelve-Sutra process is not complete until we make a conscious effort to address our karmic deficits.

An amend suggests a change, reparation, or correction. An amend is more than "sorry." It is *prayschit—to take an action to make up for the wrong*. In other words, to repent reduces the karmic consequences. True transformation occurs upon completion of our amends. When we make our amends honestly and sincerely, our consciousness expands and the shadowy veil of falsehood disintegrates. We bask in the light of our truth.

In Hindu mythology, Durga is the deity of victory of good over evil. She is the ultimate power inherent in all creation. Durga destroys ignorance and illusion. She carries the *shakti* energy and rides a lion. Courageous and fierce, she defeats Mahisha and his army of demons to save the world. Durga represents the natural forces that both grant life and remove it. Responsibility cultivates a dedication to preserving life because of how precious life actually is. When we take responsibility, as Durga did to overcome Mahisha and save the world, we uplift humanity. This sense of responsibility starts with our self and permeates into the greater context of the world.

Durga puja, a Hindu ritual or offering to the goddess Durga, epitomizes the victory of good over evil. Sutra Nine requires a warrior mentality to overcome darkness. We must follow through with this final cleansing sutra in order to become the best version of ourselves. In the Hindu epic *Mahabharata*, Lord Shiva creates a fierce warrior from a bead of sweat on his forehead. The warrior's name is *Virabhadra*. In yoga, *virabhadrasana II*, or warrior II, is the embodiment of concentrated might. In this posture, you embody a mighty conqueror willing to take on any opponent.

The conscious action necessary for this sutra relies on our level of Self-realization, or awareness. We are being guided by the innate intelligence and wisdom within that becomes accessible when we clear our negative karma. This is our nature and our truth. Swami Chidbavananda comments on the Bhagavad Gita:

"The more one attunes one's mind to the truth, the more one gains in equilibrium. The truth is, the lord is the invisible propeller of all actions in the universe. He is the true owner of everything sentient and insentient. Man's prerogative is to know this truth and adjust his life activities accordingly."[1]

Timing is Crucial

In Sutra Nine, we take action but do not become concerned with the results of our actions. In chapter two, of the Bhagavad Gita, Krishna tells Arjuna, "You have a right to perform your prescribed duty, but you are not entitled to the fruits of action. Never consider yourself the cause of the results of your activities, and never be attached to not doing your duty."[2] Pravritti—steady, consistent action—is needed for Sutra Nine. But within that action, knowing when to surrender is equally important. Proper timing is crucial when making amends.

I have found through my own amends process that the universe will place people in my path at the most appropriate time. At one point, I was procrastinating making an amend to a particular person. But everywhere I went, this person happened to be. I would go to the grocery store and see her and I would attempt to walk by without her noticing, but we ran into each other at the exit. A few weeks later, I ran in to her again. It was as if the universe was leading me to my assignment. I couldn't ignore it anymore. I had to make the amend.

More than making the actual verbal amend, we must take action not to repeat the same harm. It's our generous efforts and acts of kindness that speak to people. It's not necessarily what we are saying but, rather, who we are being and how we are behaving. Therefore, when taking action, I surrender and have patience and trust that a Higher Power is in control and the outcome will depend on my willingness to merge into a co-creating partnership with this guiding force. We are merely tourists on the divine tour bus.

I always find that I enjoy car rides more when I am relaxed and allow the driver to be in control. Self-will is attempting to be the backseat driver. We are not in control, yet we feel the need to exert some sort of authority over the situation. For addicted individuals, it is this "self-will run riot" that takes us off our path.

I noticed this often when riding in the car with my mother. She would set the destination in the navigation system, but she invariably ended up following her own directions. The GPS would guide us to make a left turn, but she would decide to turn right, thinking her directions would get us to the destination faster. It was humorous to observe her doing this. Why use a GPS then? A GPS (Guru Protection Service) never fails, in my experience.

Heeding Divine Messages

Reflecting on my past, I perceived when the universe was truly trying to get my attention. I wasn't willing to surrender and heed the "ominous warnings," as the *Big Book of Alcoholics Anonymous* calls them. A few years ago, I had become involved in a potential whistle-blower case at a previous job. As I was trying to fax a contract to the law firm handling the case, I got a call that the fax machine at their end would be down for several hours. Intuitively, it occurred to me that I probably should not follow through with the accusation. I ended up making amends to my company for my involvement, and later was summoned to testify, but I could have prevented the whole situation if I had followed divine guidance in the first place.

Now, It's Your Turn:

This is one of the most difficult of the Twelve Sutras. So, referring to your list from Sutra Eight, first imagine the entire scenario of making amends to a particular person you've harmed.

1) Find a quiet spot to sit for at least five minutes:
2) Envision yourself approaching this person, explaining that you know you've caused him/her harm, and that you want to make amends to make things right. What would you say? How would you respond? Send them love and light.
3) Then after you have played out this exchange in your mind, approach him/her in person and make your amends. Notice how the actual encounter plays out differently than you imagined. Maybe your concerns about the encounter were out of proportion to the encounter itself. Whatever the case may be, don't judge the outcome. Your access to power lies in taking 100% responsibility.
4) You have accomplished your goal, now move ahead. Continue this process for everyone on your eighth-sutra list.

A true amend is the willingness we display to show up and take responsibility for our shortcomings. The *Twelve and Twelve* states, "For the readiness to take the full consequences of our past acts, and to take responsibility for the well-being of others at the same time, is the very spirit of Step Nine."[3] With this acknowledgment comes freedom to live fully in the present, "clearing away the wreckage of our past," as noted in the *Big Book of Alcoholics Anonymous*. Action is necessary for miraculous manifestation. The future becomes a broad, open space for pure possibility. The universal horizon opens up, as it has been patiently waiting for us to claim our divine purpose and share our gifts and talents with others.

SUTRA TEN

DEITY: Vishnu

PRINCIPLE: Commitment

MANTRA: *Om Namo Narayanaya*
(Chanted to invoke Vishnu's pervading power of mercy and goodness. The mantra of peace bringing balance and harmony to the world.)

ASANA: *Chakrasana* (full-wheel pose)

MEDITATION: Find a quiet spot to sit with your eyes closed for five minutes. Repeat ten times silently.

"Standing firmly on this path, I am guided back."

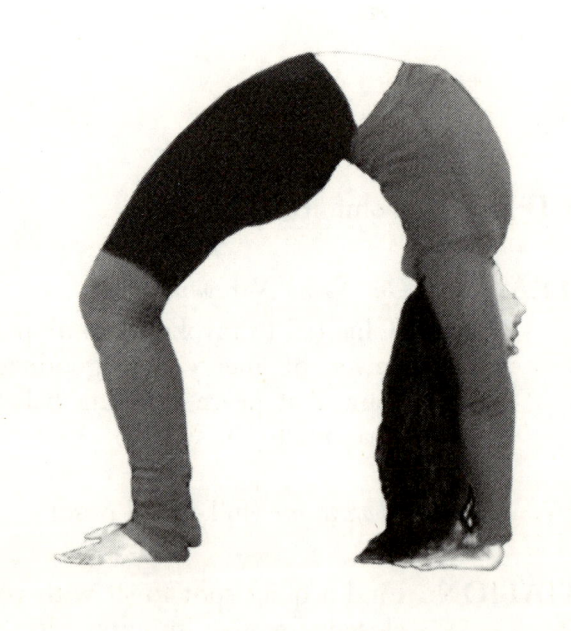

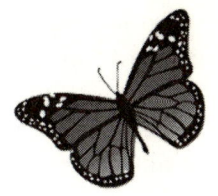

Sutra Ten: Commitment

Continue to take personal inventory and when I deviate from Love, promptly restore myself to Love.

SutraTen suggests the principle of commitment. We must become fully committed to our recovery and the personal process of Self-development. Now that we have built a foundation for a new life in Sutras One through Nine, we must continue to preserve the framework. In the cycle of life, we move through several phases and each are governed by a particular energy.

Shakti is the creative manifesting energy that underlies the universe. There are three types of Shakti, or energy: *Brahma Shakti*, the creation energy; *Vishnu Shakti*, the maintenance or preservation energy; and *Shiva Shakti*, the energy associated with destruction or dissolution. Sutra Ten illuminates the Vishnu Shakti. Vishnu is the preserver and is said to have reincarnated in times of need to bring righteousness back to humanity. Vishnu's vehicle is Garuda, the sun eagle taken from Surya. Commitment can be interpreted as dedication to a cause. In Vishnu's case, he was committed to upholding the virtues of the land, and he sought to restore them when lost. Commitment is a pledge to align yourself to a purpose or cause, come what may.

Addicted individuals have a tendency to rise very quickly and fall just as hard. In active addiction, we may lack commitment when it comes to staying the course. In Ayurveda, addiction is primarily an imbalance in the Vata dosha (prana vayu) and Vata rules movement. When Vata is high, grounded-ness and stability are lacking. Vata types will be very determined for a short period of time. Sutra Ten, or a daily inventory, keeps us practical, focused, and disciplined–all qualities contrary to those that drove us during our active addiction.

Addicted individuals may be brilliant minds, dynamic personalities, and creative geniuses. Yet after we lay the initial groundwork, we tend to rest on our laurels for the follow-through.

My nine years in and out of recovery were a continuous phoenix process, in which I would rise to a certain level of success and achievement and then burn myself into ashes of self-destruction. This course of action is mentally and emotionally draining and eventually the consequences become more and more severe. Addiction can catapult us from joy to jail in a matter of seconds. Carefully and proactively monitoring our actions, motives, and behaviors on a daily basis is a necessary preventive measure.

A Daily Karmic Spot Check

Sutra Ten is our daily karmic spot check. This is the first of the maintenance sutras. As addicted individuals, we are good at creating and destroying, but sometimes lack the daily, consistent effort necessary to sustain and maintain our recovery. Sutra Ten requires daily self-reflection and analysis.

Self-inquiry becomes valuable in this sutra. In Sanskrit we call self-inquiry *atman-vichara,* which means constant analysis of the "I-thought," in order to differentiate between the "I" (or the ego) and the Self (or the Higher Self). Through constant analysis of our life, we are able to identify the motivating factors behind our actions and behaviors. Our intentions are illuminated. When we act in accordance with love (our true nature), we accumulate karmic credit. When we listen to our ego and react on its behalf, we rack up karmic debt. Atman-vichara is a tool to analyze our karmic debts. Maintaining credit in any account—financial or spiritual—is necessary to sustain ourselves. One scripture states,

"Enquiry should be made this wise: With the kind of help of the Sat Guru one should enquire 'Who am I? What is this world? What is the reality behind all this?'"[1]

A personal inventory is a complete self-analysis, surveying our actions, behaviors, and thoughts. It requires us to maintain our physical, emotional, mental, and spiritual stability, which is the foundation for our recovery. A personal inventory is a daily housecleaning. In the fourth sutra, we conducted a thorough housecleaning, often getting into the cracks and crevices that had not been uncovered in quite some time. We cleansed our minds of negativity, fears, and resentments that kept us disconnected from ourselves and our divine nature.

By practicing a daily tenth sutra, we maintain our serenity by attending to our thoughts, actions, and deeds, and acknowledging when we may have strayed from divine guidance. A personal inventory allows us to review our day and assess how we handled our interactions with people and situations. We can reflect on where we acted consciously, with mindfulness, and where we may have fallen short. Acting consciously means being aware that what we say and do in any given situation will have an effect—positive or negative. For every action, there is an equal and opposite karmic reaction.

In the tenth sutra, we can create a safeguard to prevent our character defects from resurfacing. *Promptly admitting our wrongs* refers to making an honest appraisal of ourselves and admitting when we may have acted outside our own moral parameters. This sutra literally allows us to "keep our side of the street clean," as spoken about in Twelve Step programs.

Through the process of working the Twelve Sutras, we become accountable and responsible. Part of that process is managing our own character and being aware of how we present that character to others. In this sutra, we reduce our chances of producing more undesirable karma. This sutra is an internal karmic tracking device that we can access and adjust as we move throughout our day. We can continuously check in with ourselves and observe our thoughts, emotions, and behaviors.

Now, It's Your Turn:

Note: Sutra Ten is meant to be completed at the end of the day. First, start to observe the effects produced by your actions and notice if they are generating harmony or discord.

Daily Karmic Spreadsheet:

<u>Karmic Merits (Acts of Love)</u>   <u>Demerits (Acts of Fear)</u>

Next, take an honest inventory of your day:

1) Have you been kind and compassionate to others?
2) Have you been critical?
3) Are you being honest with yourself about your motives?
4) Are your motives fear-based or love-based?
5) Have you acted out of alignment with your Higher Power?
6) Have you expressed love in all your daily encounters?
7) Are you enhancing the lives of others around you or are your behaviors menacing?

Be specific, and in situations where you have fallen short, promptly admit that to yourself and to those your actions may have harmed.

In Alcoholics Anonymous, members understand they have a "daily reprieve contingent upon the maintenance of our spiritual condition."[2] Sutra Ten is a measuring gauge for our spiritual condition. Just as a barometer measures the air pressure, which fluctuates throughout the day, Sutra Ten measures our fluctuating spiritual climate. We must acknowledge our assets and liabilities on a daily basis. Consistent observation of our mental patterns is a necessary part of this sutra.

Sutra Ten brings us back to a state of equilibrium. We clean up our daily karmic wreckage in order to create a pure space where Divinity can guide us toward positive action. If we go for days and weeks without cleaning our house, allowing the dust to accumulate, we begin to feel uncomfortable residing in that space. Similarly, when we neglect our own internal housecleaning, we begin to feel ill at ease.

Addicted individuals already have a tendency to feel "restless, irritable, and discontented,"[3] as noted in the *Big Book of Alcoholics Anonymous*. An addicted individual's mind naturally gravitates toward the past, triggering uncomfortable emotions, such as resentment, guilt, shame, and remorse. I was once in the emergency room with a client who had relapsed and had an extremely high blood alcohol content. She had been held up at gunpoint by a male aggressor several years before and was in a continual state of fear around men. Even in the emergency room, she was fearful of the male nurses and doctors. Her past trauma was keeping her a prisoner in the present and was also contributing to her alcohol abuse. Until she could heal her past, she would not be able to completely move forward and live a joyful, peace-filled life.

In yoga, the posture *chakrasana*, or full-wheel pose, is a cleansing tonic for the body and mind. As the body bends backwards, blood rushes to the head, clearing away anxiety and stresses in the mind and leaving us feeling invigorated. An empty mind, free of thoughts from the past, is an effective mind. With an empty space, we have the freedom to create.

Life only unfolds in the present moment; therefore, if we want to truly live in the present moment, we must rectify any and all matters that keep us disconnected from Source. We may think that we have many problems, but all our problems stem from one: our separation from Higher Consciousness.

Fear versus Love

When we create a spreadsheet and analyze our karmic assets and liabilities, we see that our liabilities have often originated as a reaction to fear, whereas our assets stem from love. We can differentiate between these two opposing energies, which are two sides of the same coin. The mind tends to focus on the liabilities or deficiencies. We may receive ten compliments and one criticism, but our mind will most likely dwell on the criticism. Critical self-analysis can lead to overkill. Fear-based thoughts will perpetuate fear-based actions and reactions, adding to our karmic deficits.

By contrast, thoughts emanating from a space of love will produce corresponding karmic merit. Enlightenment is simply the journey back to love. It is the return to who we really are and what remains constant in this universe. We will always be directed to return to what is real.

The power of love is the ultimate source of communion between everyone and everything. When we return to the present moment, we return to love. For when we are truly living, we are fearlessly loving. Love is the dynamic expression of life in the present moment, which is all there truly is.

SUTRA ELEVEN

DEITY: Saraswati

PRINCIPLE: Liberation

MANTRA: *Sarswatyai Namah*
(Salutations to the mother of knowledge)

ASANA: *Utkata Konasana* (goddess pose)

MEDITATION: Find a quiet spot. Close your eyes and repeat silently for five minutes:

"When freedom is attained, I neither want nor gain."

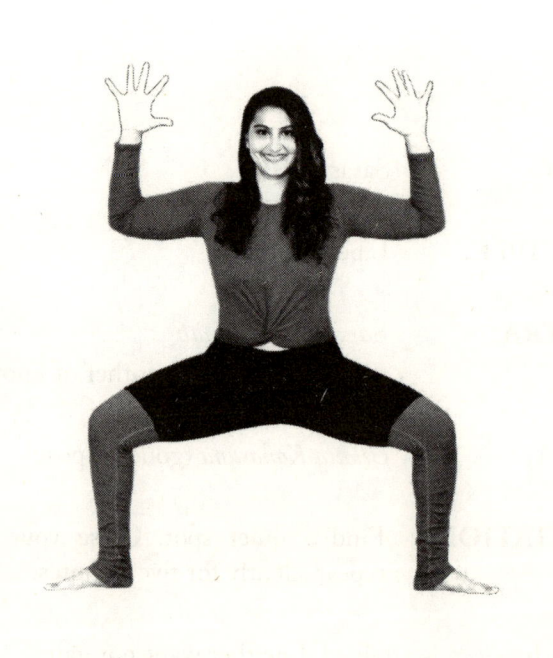

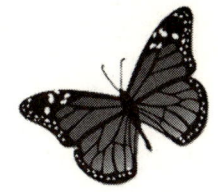

Sutra Eleven: Liberation

Seek through prayer and meditation to improve conscious contact with the Divine, as I understand the Divine, praying for knowledge of Thy will and the Power to carry it out.

God-consciousness can be awakened by purifying your system through mindfulness practices such as Sudarshan Kriya, yoga, and meditation. Step Eleven in the *Twelve Steps and Twelve Traditions* elaborates:

"When we refuse air, light, or food, the body suffers. And when we turn away from meditation and prayer, we likewise deprive our minds, our emotions, and our intuitions of vitally needed support. As the body can fail its purpose for lack of nourishment, so can the soul."[1]

Addiction is a spiritual malady that requires a spiritual remedy. It is a spiritual deficiency that calls for spiritual nourishment. When most of us come into recovery, we are spiritually starved. The nourishment that sustains us is found through prayer and meditation.

Prayer and meditation are an addicted individual's soul food. Meditation is our direct connection to the Source, or Divinity, and activates the innate intelligence that resides at our very core. Meditation is creativity's midwife. We possess gifts that lay dormant but can be uncovered, discovered, and nurtured through meditation. While in our mother's womb, we were in a state of meditation. For nine months, we were in a state of *samadhi*, the state of integration and wholeness, until being born into this physical world. In meditation, we return to that quiet, undisturbed space of solitude. We repose into ourselves.

As a recovered individual, this is the only productive form of escape I have ever known. Trying to escape life by abusing toxic substances made my life unbalanced and compromised my health. Addicted individuals seek a transcendent experience. Drugs and alcohol may bring on that heightened state of being or altered state of consciousness temporarily, but eventually the "chase" to re-create the experience produces detrimental effects in our lives.

I remember being in detox unit for a Klonopin addiction and a girl asked me if I had ever "chased the dragon." Apparently, she was referring to smoking heroin. It later occurred to me that what I was actually chasing was always present within me. In reality, I had been "chasing the guru." I had been yearning to experience my own Divinity. The guru is a mirror that reflects our own divine nature. Meditation illuminates our Divinity or God-consciousness, allowing it to radiate outwards. There is a section in the Bhagavad Gita that states, "With the Self detached from the external contacts he realizes the bliss in the Self. Devoted as he is to the meditation of Brahman, he enjoys imperishable Bliss."[2]

Addiction to Bliss

This bliss, or *ananda* in Sanskrit, is intoxicating. Addiction to bliss is "chasing the guru." But what we are truly addicted to is our complete connection to the love within ourselves and the love we experience when ego diminishes and we connect to Brahman, or the "One," the all-pervading force. We dissolve into the abundant field of love that surrounds us. This ecstasy can be accessed through meditation or conscious contact with Divinity. When we empty all thoughts of who we think we are, we become an empty vessel for divine inspiration. Meditation will provide us with all the answers and guidance we are seeking because all the answers to our questions lie within us.

I remember being on the ninth sutra and I was sitting in meditation one day. All of a sudden I recalled an amend I needed to make. The amend was not on my original list. I was not able to consciously access the amend with my intellect alone, but through meditation I was provided with the appropriate information at exactly the right time.

When we work the Twelve Sutras, a psychic change or internal shift occurs. We have cleared away the darkness, allowing the light to shine forth. Therefore, consciously working the Twelve Sutras is a spiritual practice, but we must go deeper; we must access our Divinity and allow our true nature to blossom. *The Twelve Steps and Twelve Traditions* elaborates on this in Step Eleven:

"We will want the good that is in us all, even in the worst of us, to flower and to grow. Most certainly we shall need bracing air and an abundance of food. But first of all we shall want sunlight; nothing much can grow in the dark. Meditation is our step out into the sun."[3]

Throughout our active addiction, we engineer patterns of behavior that are usually detrimental to our existence. These patterns leave encryptions in the subtle body, known as *samskaras*. Meditation eliminates samskaras which, in turn, eliminate negative karma. The more you meditate, the more you free yourself from the past, accelerating your spiritual advancement.

The Purpose of Meditation

Meditation clarifies knowledge of Source's will and the power to carry it out. It is the very medium that brings this power to the surface and infuses our life with ultimate wisdom. Wisdom lies in the "knowing," or resting in the ultimate, expansive presence of life.

Meditation is the silent communication of the universe's will for us. Sometimes what cannot be heard through our limited senses can be transmitted through direct experience. Aligning ourselves with the present moment through meditation enables us to live expansively and magnify the possibility contained in each opportunity we encounter. We gradually move back into the inner world, nivritti, or embracing the Self.

I was a short-distance sprinter in high school and I once had an experience after running the 100-meter dash. I remember the gun going off and for twelve seconds, I was completely detached from my surroundings. After I crossed the finish line, my friends and family asked if I heard them cheering me on from the sidelines. I was so lost in the experience of the race that I hadn't heard anything. That twelve seconds of pure nivritti was a moving meditation.

Now, It's Your Turn:

Sobering Samadhi:

1) Think back to a time when you were sober, aware, and felt completely immersed in the present moment, in the "flow" of life. Describe this experience in detail. Write down as much about this experience as you can.

2) Now close your eyes and for five minutes access those feelings. Imagine the vitality of that experience and bring it in to this moment.

3) When you open your eyes, allow the bliss you have generated to permeate your body.

Repeat this exercise as often as you like.

Prayer versus Meditation

Prayer is as much a daily spiritual practice as meditation. Prayer is communicating with a Higher Power and meditation is becoming the empty receptacle to receive spiritual guidance. When we pray for "knowledge of Thy will for us," we are praying for signs and confirmation that we are on the right path, that our actions and motives are born from a place of purity and love. In prayer, the Divine's will, essentially merges with our will.

I remember asking a spiritual mentor and NYT best-selling author, Gabrielle Bernstein, how to differentiate between God's will and my will. She replied, "Let it all be God's will."

Our will, our wants, our desires, and our needs, born from the "I-thought," no longer hold any significance when we embark on the spiritual path. In the program of Alcoholics Anonymous, it is said that God is either everything or nothing. Understanding that all of humanity is connected and that Divinity dwells in this entire creation leads us to liberation or freedom from samsara, worldly existence.

The Goal of Liberation

No amount of pleasure from the external world will satisfy the desire for security. Freedom, or liberation from worldly bondage, is called *moksha* in Sanskrit. As we near completion of the Twelve Sutras, we abandon prior pursuits and devote ourselves to fulfilling our soulful purpose and carrying out our dharmic responsibility. Swami Dayananda captures this transition beautifully:

"So, when a mature person analyses his experiences, he discovers that behind his pursuit of security and pleasure is a basic desire to be free from all insufficiency, to be free from incompleteness itself, a basic desire which no amount of *artha* and *kama* fulfills. This realization brings a certain dispassion, *nirveda*, towards security and pleasures. The mature person gains dispassion towards his former pursuits and is ready to seek liberation, *moksha*, directly."[4]

A seeker of moksha, or an informed seeker, is known as a *mumuksu*. A mumuksu knows that he is both the seeker and the possessor. The adequacy he seeks is not separate from himself and is not to be obtained through efforts or exertion. The end is inherent in the means and the realization of this becomes apparent through destruction of ignorance and Self-actualization. Meditation dissolves this ignorance, making the truth attainable.

In Hindu mythology, many people worship the deity *Saraswati* to be granted moksha. She is often depicted as a beautiful woman seated on a white swan, symbolizing that she is rooted in the experience of absolute truth. She wears a mala of crystals, representing the power of meditation and spirituality. Saraswati's color is white, symbolic of peace. Her companion is a white Swan.

The Swan is a symbol of purity, beauty, grace, love and elegance, but it can also symbolize divination and balance.

Liberation from bondage of the material world leads to internal peace. Inward-focused practices, such as yoga, Sudarshan Kriya, and meditation are tools to accessing this peace, love, and grace. Seek to move inward. In yoga, the posture *utkata konasana*, or goddess pose, exemplifies reverence to the goddess. In a squatted position, the chest is upright with the palms in a prayer position at the center of the heart, acknowledging attunement to the truth. According to the *Twelve Steps and Twelve Traditions:*

"Perhaps one of the greatest rewards of meditation and prayer is the sense of belonging that comes to us. The moment we catch even a glimpse of God's will, the moment we begin to see truth, justice, and love as the real and eternal things in life, we are no longer deeply disturbed by all the seeming evidence to the contrary that surrounds us in purely human affairs."[5]

SUTRA TWELVE

DEITY: Krishna

PRINCIPLE: Dharma

MANTRA: *Om Krishnaya Namahah*
(O Lord Krishna, I salute you, the road to dharma)

ASANA: *Virasana* (hero's pose)

MEDITATION: Sit quietly for five minutes. Close your eyes and repeat ten times:

"From ashes I rise, dutiful and wise."

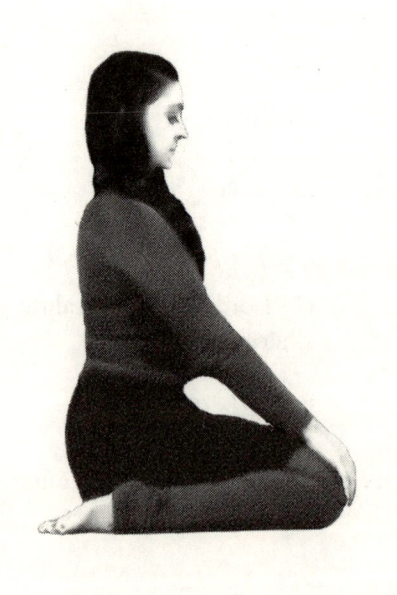

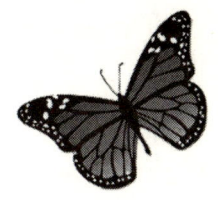

Sutra Twelve: Dharma

Having had a spiritual awakening as the result of these Sutras, I carry this message to others, and practice these Sutras in all worldly affairs.

Spiritual awakening

A revolutionary shift in thought and perception supported through an intimate experience and connection with a Power greater than our finite selves. A shift in consciousness from fixation and immersion in maya (illusion) to an expanded state of awareness linked to a connection with our inner Divinity.

We are spiritual beings having a human experience so we strive to live without attachment to maya, or the illusory physical manifestation of form. We use the Twelve Sutras as a practical guide to living life most effectively in the physical plane but being careful not to get drawn into the illusion. All physical matter—everything our senses perceive—is an illusion. Deepak Chopra points out that what is experienced through our senses or imagination isn't actually "Real" in the true sense and in forgetting the "Real," humans create illusions. This relates to the Hindu notion of "maya." We perceive that the sensory inputs are real, but our divine intelligence is connected to a higher realm. Every "thing" carries a vibration or current of energy and it is this energy that attracts or repels. This is the realm of infinite creation.

The observer is our "wise self," Jung's archetypal "wise old man." The observer resides in the "gap," as Deepak Chopra calls it.

Let the gap be your home base but stay close to the realm of Higher Consciousness. Your spiritual body is your true Self. Your physical body is simply an instrument to carry out your dharma, or duty, in the physical world. Do not get caught up in the neurosis and mania of activity in the physical world.

Maya yoga (yoga means "union") can relate to union with the illusion and attachment to the nonreal. It is very alluring, even addictive at times, because the ego is caught in the separation from our true Self or spiritual essence.

Have you ever been in a conversation and just stepped back and observed what is being said? If you listen closely, it sometimes resembles an egoic dance party. Learn to listen for the intention behind the words–the unspoken communication. Pay attention to the process, not the content. When you are able to do this consistently, your intuition will develop. Ask yourself, "What is my dharma in this conversation?" Maybe your purpose is simply to observe and not engage. Every second is an opportunity for learning. Be open-minded. Accept crisis, for with it comes opportunity. Your life will unfold in front of you the more you get to know, love, and understand yourself. As Shakespeare said, "To thine own self be true."

The Three Spiritual Components

We all have three spiritual components: a student, a teacher, and a master. Each becomes more pronounced during different periods of our life.

We begin as a student in all areas of our life. We take in information, assimilate it, and apply it to our life. Step by step, we gain knowledge about particular subjects. We take in what resonates and we discard the rest. This is the beginning of our journey. Soon we find a topic that sparks our interest and we make a subtle commitment to delve into it. Then we seek out teachers who provide us with information or knowledge to nurture our desire to progress. As our commitment grows stronger, the energy moves in that direction and more people come into our life who will support us. This is growth. We are essentially nurturing the seed, watering it, and allowing it to sprout. But we realize that our growth in that area depends on sharing what we have learned. We want to put what we have learned into practice.

So we move into the next phase: We teach what we have learned. We test our strengths. In this phase, do not be concerned with the audience. You may initially only have two students. Your purpose in this phase is to experiment and learn.

When I first began teaching yoga, I had a very small class of only two or three students. I was more concerned with mastering my teaching skills than building my class size. As you refine your craft, the people who will benefit will arrive. Use the knowledge you have and your own creativity to share what you have learned but, go about it with the intention to serve. Become more attuned to the experience. You will have time to evaluate later. Be present with your experience. In order for others to respond to your teachings, become part of their experience. Give 100 percent to them and then watch what unfolds!

I have always been an avid exerciser, and in my early twenties I started attending a variety of fitness classes. I took classes from a broad range of teachers, gaining insights from different styles of exercises, such as kickboxing, aqua aerobics, and step aerobics. Eventually, my interest became so strong that I wanted to become a teacher. When I became certified and started teaching classes at several gyms, I fine-tuned my skills even more. I was developing my own routines and had found an outlet for my creativity. As a result, I became a successful fitness instructor at a number of gyms as well as a private instructor. Where there is dedication, there is success.

We who are on the spiritual path have a responsibility to gather others and bring them along. We are on this journey together. Suffering begins when we see each other as separate from ourselves. In reality, we are all one.

Only when you become tired of being bound to an illusion will you awaken to your truest potential. You have a responsibility to share your gifts with the world. There are sick and suffering souls who are lost, and you may be able to help them. Keep your eyes directed on the inner beauty and your external world will be filled with beauty. Have a mustard seed of willingness to seek, because the knowledge is endless, but everything begins with yourself. Create for others what you wish for yourself. But be aware that you must nourish yourself before you can sustain others. It will always begin with you and it will always end with you.

You have everything you need to live the life you have always imagined. But your vision must be clear and your intentions pure. Abusing any substance to fix a problem is simply applying a Band-Aid remedy. It is like filling potholes rather than repaving the street. If you can learn to build something solid, which may require more time, effort, and resources in the short term, this will inevitably produce lasting results in the long term.

That is what *sustainability* means. If we can build a more sustainable society, we have a better chance of forging a harmonious society in which all species coexist and benefit from each other. Life on earth is symbiotic, interdependent. We are each other's greatest assets.

Our Purpose: Service

The virtue of Sutra Twelve is service, or *seva*. It is essential for recovering addicted individuals to maintain their recovery through selfless service to others. The obsession with self, or asmita, creates the suffering, and the solution lies in the dissolution of asmita, or focusing away from self through seva. Because we live on the material, physical plane, and surviving requires gains, we have a tendency to become attached to our own wants and needs. When our time and energy are devoted to satisfying our self, we lose focus on the wider lens of why we are here: to fulfill our dharma. We have all chosen this lifetime for a specific purpose, and only because of the unique nature of our individual talents and gifts are we able to fulfill our dharma. A life lived without recognizing and embracing our dharma becomes futile. A mind focused on dharma in all aspects of life, in all situations, is at ease.

Fulfilling dharma, or duty, is the principal means of gaining liberation. Purposeful action with spiritually sound motives dispels negative karma and bondage. As the Maharishi notes:

"Dharma is that invincible power of nature which upholds existence. It maintains evolution and forms the very basis of cosmic life. It supports all that is helpful for evolution and discourages all that is opposed to it. Dharma is that which promotes worldly prosperity and spiritual freedom."[1]

Aligning with Our Dharma

When we are in alignment with our dharma, life becomes effortless. I always felt that it was my dharma to write because I had a message to convey and I knew there was an audience that would benefit from the message. I never recognized the value of the challenges I faced throughout my life until I began using them as a means to help others.

Our ultimate dharma in every circumstance is to be of maximum service. Even Alcoholics Anonymous suggests that our primary purpose is to "carry the message." We cannot truly keep it unless we give it away–and continue to give it away for the rest of our lives. We do not evolve on the spiritual path unless we help others find where theirs begins.

Now, It's Your Turn:

Come up with one service initiative of your own design. Be creative. Find a way to enhance your community. One small act can go a long way. Here are a few examples:

1) Donate clothes to a homeless shelter or a recovery home.
2) Offer to walk a dog at your local animal shelter.
3) Bake cookies for residents of a nursing home.

There is no limit to how much you can light up this world! Shine brightly for someone today!

The soul of recovery is service. It is the backbone of our existence. When we are fully established in our dharma and focused on the higher evolution of humanity, all our wants and needs seem to be effortlessly fulfilled.

As I was writing this book, the universe was supporting me from all angles. I would often find inspiration from other books that would literally be placed in my lap or given to me at exactly the right time. I would find myself spontaneously conversing with editors or other aspiring writers. In fact, just prior to the actual publication, I had queried over 30 agents and publishers. To my surprise, when I let go and trusted that the pieces would come together in Divine timing, I received an email from a publisher, who ended up being the exact fit for this book. My world was arranging itself according to the Divine plan, enabling me to fulfill my dharma.

Fulfilling our dharma promotes progression on the spiritual path. Why remain stagnant in this world? Life in human form is precious. When we honor what we have come here to do, all the guilt and shame surrounding our past addiction becomes nonexistent. There is no higher calling than honoring our dharma, carrying it out, and being of maximum service to the Divine.

In the Bhagavad Gita, Krishna reveals to Arjuna the essence of selfless action. Krishna exclaims, "Surrendering all your actions unto Me, your thoughts concentrated on the Absolute, free from selfishness and without anticipation of reward, with mind devoid of excitement—fight!"[2] Krishna emphasizes to Arjuna the importance of carrying out his dharma. Krishna later tells Arjuna that he has nothing to fear because divine protection is always with him. The Bhagavad Gita is considered to be the "gospel" of Hinduism. In it, Krishna promises to defeat evil and deliver piousness to the descendants of Bharata. Part of Krishna's dharma is to be a warrior and fight. It was his assigned role on the earthly realm. Fulfillment of dharma was his ultimate goal.

In Sanskrit, the yoga pose *virasana*, is also called "hero's pose." Heroes and heroines often experience obstacles and setbacks before they win their battles. In Jungian psychology, the hero archetype is also known as the warrior, crusader, or soldier. The goal of the hero archetype is to achieve mastery in a way that improves the world.

Every conversation you have with another person is a dharmic assignment. It is an opportunity to be an agent of love. Keep an open mind and ask yourself, "What is my dharma in this moment?" The *Twelve Steps and Twelve Traditions* notes, "And then he discovers that by the divine paradox of this kind of giving he has found his own reward, whether his brother has yet received anything or not."[3]

You can always choose the higher path, and when you do, everyone benefits.

Conclusion

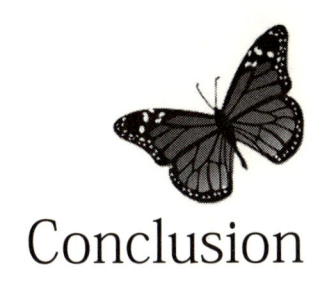

And so, my dear friends, we have reached the end of our journey together. But remember, that every ending is a predestined new beginning. You have just begun to climb the mountain toward your destiny. As you embrace your newfound path to recovery, remember that it will always lead you home. When life's challenges and disappointments occur, honor them as an opportunity to grow into the highest version of yourself. Lean into the hardship, for the crisis is always the opportunity, and above all, do not sacrifice your Self. Sacrifice your fear.

I leave you with one last powerful mantra:

Asato Ma Sad Gamaya
Tamaso Ma Jyotir Gamaya
Mrityor Ma Anritam Gamaya

Lead me from the unreal to the Real
Lead me from the darkness to the Light
Lead me from the temporary to the Eternal

Namaste.

Glossary

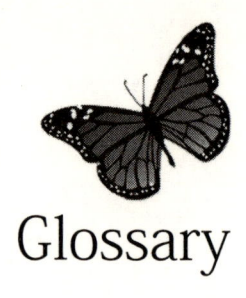

Akasha: the space element, ether, the basis of all creation

Ananda: happiness, bliss

Anitya: impermanent, transient

Asmita: egoism

Atman: Self

Atma-vichara: self-evaluation

Avidya: ignorance

Bhagavad: divine

Brahma Jnanam: Divine or sacred Self-knowledge

Brahmin: someone who is immersed in Brahma-gyan or knowledge of the Divine.

Dharma: duty

Dosha: (in Ayurvedic medicine) each of three energies which circulate in the body and govern physiological activity.

Gita: song

Guna: quality

Guru: teacher

Jeeva: individual(soul)

Kama: desire

Karma: action

Krodha: anger

Lobha: greed

Mada: passion

Matsarya: jealousy

Maya: world of unreality or illusion

Moha: delusion

Moksha: liberation

Mumuksu: a seeker of *moksha*, or liberation

Nivritti: inclination towards the inner world, retreat from the outer

Prakriti: nature

Prana: life force

Pravritti: inclination towards outer action or the outer world

Purusha: Self that pervades the universe

Rajasic: property of nature characterized by activity

Samadhi: deep state of meditation

Samsara: worldly existence

Samskara: impression

Sankalpa: intention

Sattva: property of nature characterized by goodness, purity

Seva: service

Shakti: energy

Spiritual awakening: A revolutionary shift in thought and perception supported through an intimate experience and connection with a Power greater than our finite selves. A shift in consciousness from fixation and immersion in *maya* (the world of illusion) to an expanded state of awareness linked to a connection with our inner Divinity.

Sudarshan kriya: a rhythmic breathing and detoxification technique discovered by Sri Sri Ravi Shankar and taught by The Art of Living Foundation

Tamasic: property of nature characterized by darkness, dullness

Tattva: principle, truth, reality

Veda: knowledge

Vedanta: complete knowledge of the Upanishads, the end of the Veda

Yoga: union

Shraddha: faith

Notes

Preface

1. Carl Jung, *Man and His Symbols* (London: Aldus Books, 1968), p. 169.

Introduction

1. William R. Miller, Alyssa A. Forcehimes, and Allen Zweben, *Treating Addiction: A Guide for Professionals* (New York: Guilford Press, 2011), p. 71.

Sutra One

1. *Bhagavad Gita.* https://www.goodreads.com/quotes/1394795-you-have-the-right-to-work-but-for-the-work-s (accessed December 15, 2019).
2. Sampananda Mishra, "Two Paths: Shreyas and Preyas." http://bhagavadgita.org.in/Blogs/5ab0b9b75369ed21c4c74c01 (accessed December 15, 2019).
3. Alcoholics Anonymous. "A.A. Timeline." http://www.aa.org/pages/en_US/aa-timeline (accessed June 13, 2014).
4. Lynn W. White, "Recovery from Alcoholism: Transpersonal Dimensions," *Journal of Transpersonal Psychology* 11, no. 2 (1979): pp. 117–128.
5. Lynn W. White, "Recovery from Alcoholism: Transpersonal Dimensions," *Journal of Transpersonal Psychology* 11, no. 2 (1979): 64.

Sutra Two

1. Swami Chinmayananda. *Vedanta: The Science of Life* (Mumbai: Triumph Press Pvt. Ltd, 1983), p. 190.
2. Swami Chinmayananda. *Vedanta: The Science of Life* (Mumbai: Triumph Press Pvt. Ltd, 1983), p. 183.

Sutra Three

1. Swami Chinmayananda. *Vedanta: The Science of Life* (Mumbai: Triumph Press Pvt. Ltd, 1983), p. 191.
2. RumiShams.com. *Rumi and Shams: The Eternal Friendship.* http://www.rumishams.com/home.html (accessed January 21, 2021).
3. Helen Schucman and William Thetford, *A Course in Miracles*, (Mill Valley: Foundation for Inner Peace, 2007), p. T-25.I.7:1.
4. *Ibid.*
5. Swami Chinmayananda. *Vedanta: The Science of Life* (Mumbai: Triumph Press Pvt. Ltd, 1983), p. 126.
6. Swami Chinmayananda. *Vedanta: The Science of Life* (Mumbai: Triumph Press Pvt. Ltd, 1983), p. 125.
7. Bill Wilson. *The Big Book of Alcoholics Anonymous* (New York: Alcoholics Anonymous, 2001), p. 20.

Sutra Four

1. Brian Weiss, MD. *Through Time Into Healing: How Past Life Regression Therapy Can Heal Mind, Body and Soul* (London: Piatkus, 2013), p. 122.
2. Swami Chinmayananda. *Vedanta: The Science of Life* (Mumbai: Triumph Press Pvt. Ltd, 1983), p. 105.
3. Narcotics Anonymous. *Narcotics Anonymous* (Chatsworth: NA World Services, 2008), p. 50.
4. Swami Chidbhavananda. *The Bhagavad Gita* (Tirupparaithurai: Sri Ramakrishna Tapovanam, 2008), pp. 260-261.

Sutra Five

1. Swami Chinmayananda. *Vedanta: The Science of Life* (Mumbai: Triumph Press Pvt. Ltd, 1983), p. 17.
2. Peter Levine, PhD. *In An Unspoken Voice: How the Body Releases*

Trauma and Restores Goodness (Berkeley, CA: North Atlantic Books, 2010), p. 37.
3. Ibid.
4. Marianne Williamson. *A Return to Love.*(New York: Harper Collins, 1992), pp. 53-54.
5. Swami Chinmayananda. *Vedanta: The Science of Life* (Mumbai: Triumph Press Pvt. Ltd, 1983), p. 264.

Sutra Six

1. Swami Chinmayananda. *Vedanta: The Science of Life* (Mumbai: Triumph Press Pvt. Ltd, 1983), p. 204.
2. Swami Chidbhavananda. *The Bhagavad Gita* (Tirupparaithurai: Sri Ramakrishna Tapovanam, 2008).
3. Bill Wilson. *The Big Book of Alcoholics Anonymous* (New York: Alcoholics Anonymous, 2001), p. 62.
4. Swami Chidbhavananda. *The Bhagavad Gita* (Tirupparaithurai: Sri Ramakrishna Tapovanam, 2008), p. 300.
5. Swami Chinmayananda. *Vedanta: The Science of Life* (Mumbai: Triumph Press Pvt. Ltd, 1983), p. 199.
6. Swami Chidbhavananda. *The Bhagavad Gita* (Tirupparaithurai: Sri Ramakrishna Tapovanam, 2008), [Chapter 5, verses 16-17].
7. Swami Chinmayananda. *Vedanta: The Science of Life* (Mumbai: Triumph Press Pvt. Ltd, 1983), p. 252.

Sutra Seven

1. Charles Bates. *Ransoming the Mind* (St. Paul: Yes International Publishers, 1986), pp. 58-59.
2. Alcoholics Anonymous. *The Twelve Steps and Twelve Traditions* (New York: Alcoholics Anonymous, 2002), p. 72.
3. David Simon, MD and Deepak Chopra, MD. *Freedom From Addiction* (Deerfield Beach: Health Communications Inc., 2007), p. 36.

Sutra Eight

1. Alcoholics Anonymous. *The Twelve Steps and Twelve Traditions* (New York: Alcoholics Anonymous, 2002), p. 77.
2. Swami Vivekenanda. *Karma Yoga* (Kolkata: Advaita Ashrama, 2007), p. 53.

3. Swami Chidbhavananda. *The Bhagavad Gita* (Tirupparaithurai: Sri Ramakrishna Tapovanam, 2008), p. 211.
4. Deepak Chopra. *Overcoming Addictions.* (New York: Three Rivers Press, 1997), p. 4.
5. Helen Schucman and William Thetford, *A Course in Miracles*, (Mill Valley: Foundation for Inner Peace, 2007), p. 354.
6. Helen Schucman and William Thetford, *A Course in Miracles*, (Mill Valley: Foundation for Inner Peace, 2007), p. 357.
7. V. Ramanathan. *Ramayana For Children* (Mumbai: Giri Trading Agency, 2003), p. 170.

Sutra Nine

1. Swami Chidbhavananda. *The Bhagavad Gita* (Tirupparaithurai: Sri Ramakrishna Tapovanam, 2008), p. 252.
2. Swami Chidbhavananda. *The Bhagavad Gita* (Tirupparaithurai: Sri Ramakrishna Tapovanam, 2008).
3. Alcoholics Anonymous. *The Twelve Steps and Twelve Traditions* (New York: Alcoholics Anonymous, 2002), p. 87.

Sutra Ten

1. Sage Ribhu. *Ribhu Gita* Ch. 32, v21.
2. Bill Wilson. *The Big Book of Alcoholics Anonymous* (New York: Alcoholics Anonymous, 2001), p. 85.
3. Bill Wilson. *The Big Book of Alcoholics Anonymous* (New York: Alcoholics Anonymous, 2001), pp. xxv-xxxii.

Sutra Eleven

1. Alcoholics Anonymous. *The Twelve Steps and Twelve Traditions* (New York: Alcoholics Anonymous, 2002), p. 97.
2. Swami Chidbhavananda. *The Bhagavad Gita* (Tirupparaithurai: Sri Ramakrishna Tapovanam, 2008), p. 346.
3. Alcoholics Anonymous. *The Twelve Steps and Twelve Traditions* (New York: Alcoholics Anonymous, 2002), p. 98.
4. Swami Dayanada. *Introduction to Vedanta* (New Delhi: Vision Books, 2012), p. 29.
5. Alcoholics Anonymous. *The Twelve Steps and Twelve Traditions* (New York: Alcoholics Anonymous, 2002), p. 105.

Sutra Twelve

1. Swami Chidbhavananda. *The Bhagavad Gita* (Tirupparaithurai: Sri Ramakrishna Tapovanam, 2008); (Ch.1, v1).
2. Swami Chidbhavananda. *The Bhagavad Gita* (Tirupparaithurai: Sri Ramakrishna Tapovanam, 2008); (3:30).
3. Alcoholics Anonymous. *The Twelve Steps and Twelve Traditions* (New York: Alcoholics Anonymous, 2002), p. 109.

Bibliography

Alcoholics Anonymous. *Twelve Steps and Twelve Traditions.* New York: Alcoholics Anonymous, 2002.

Alcoholics Anonymous. "A.A. Timeline." http://www.aa.org/pages/en_US/aa-timeline (accessed June 21, 2014).

Bates, Charles. *Ransoming the Mind.* St. Paul: Yes International Publishers, 1986.

Chidbhavananda, Swami. *The Bhagavad Gita.* Tirupparaithurai: Sri Ramakrishna Tapovanam, 2008.

Chinmayananda, Swami. *Vedanta: The Science of Life.* Mumbai: Triumph Press Pvt. Ltd., 1983.

Dayananda, Swami. *Introduction to Vedanta.* New Dehli: Vision Books, 2012.

Green, Anne. P. *Principles of Ayurveda.* Hammersmith: Harper Collins, 2000.

Hemenway, Priya. *Hindu Gods.* San Francisco: Chronicle Books, 2003.

Levine, Peter. *In an Unspoken Voice: How the Body Releases Trauma and Restores Goodness.* Berkeley: North Atlantic Books, 2010.

Miller, William R., Forcehimes, Alyssa A., and Allen Zweben, A. *Treating Addiction: A Guide for Professionals.* New York: The Guildford Press, 2011.Narcotics Anonymous.

Narcotics Anonymous. Van Nuys CA: World Service Office, 2008.

Ramanathan, V. *Ramayana For Children.* Mumbai: Giri Trading Agency, 2003.

RumiShams.com. "Rumi and Shams: The Eternal Friendship." http://www.rumishams.com/home.html (accessed January 21, 2021)

Sage Ribhu. *Ribhu Gita* Ch. 32, v21.

Schucman, Helen, and Thetford, William. *A Course In Miracles.* Mill Valley: Foundation for Inner Peace, 2007.

Shapiro, Rami. *Recovery: The Twelve Steps as a Spiritual Practice.* Woodstock: Sky Lights Path Publishing, 2009.

Simon, David and Chopra, Deepak. *Freedom from Addiction.* Deerfield Beach: Health Communications Inc., 2007.

Svoboda, Robert. *Prakriti: Your Ayurvedic Constitution.* Twin Lakes: Lotus Press, 2011.

Vivekananda, Swami. *Karma Yoga.* Kolkata: Adavaita Ashrama, 2007.

Weiss, Brian. *Through Time Into Healing: How Past Life Regression Therapy can Heal Mind, Body, and Soul.* London: Piatkus, 2013.

White, Lynn. "Recovery from Alcholism: Transpersonal Dimensions." *The Journal of Transpersonal Psychology 11(2)*, 117- 128.

Williams, George, M. *Hindu Mythology.* Santa Barbara: George Williams, 2003.

Williamson, Marianne. *A Return to Love.* New York: Harper Collins, 1992.

Wilson, Bill. *Big Book of Alcoholics Anonymous.* New York: Alcoholics Anonymous, 2001.

www.mum.edu/msvs/6195 wells1html (pg 26-27).

IAHV & AOL Programs

International Association for Human Values (IAHV) and **The Art of Living Foundation (AOL)** offer a range of courses all featuring the powerful SKY practice. SKY stands for "Sudarshan Kriya Yoga," and is part of an ancient science of practices for maintaining health and expanding awareness. SKY Breath Meditation was designed by global humanitarian and spiritual teacher, Sri Sri Ravi Shankar.

The following IAHV & AOL programs address specific areas (Course description and registration information may be found on websites):

SKY Breath Meditation: https://www.artofliving.org/us-en
IAHV's cornerstone program for the general adult population

SKY Recovery Program: https://skyrecoveryprogram.org
IAHV's program for addiction/substance misuse-related issues

SKY Campus Happiness Program: https://www.skycampushappiness.org/
IAHV's program taught on university campuses geared toward the collegiate age group

Project Welcome Home Troops: https://projectwelcomehometroops.org/
IAHV's program designed to rehabilitate combat and returning veterans.

IAHV Prison Program: https://www.prisonprogram.org/
IAHV's rehabilitation program for offenders & incarcerated individuals, as well as correctional staff and victims of crime.

Sri Sri School of Yoga: https://srisrischoolofyoga.org/na/
AOL's yoga program offering 200 HR and 300 HR level trainings as well as yoga courses.

Author Contact:

yogaofrehab@gmail.com

Follow:

Website: anjalitalcherkar.com
Instagram: @anjalitalch
Facebook: https://www.facebook.com/anjalitalch
Twitter: https://twitter.com/AnjaliTalcherkr

GARUDA PRAKASHAN BOOKS

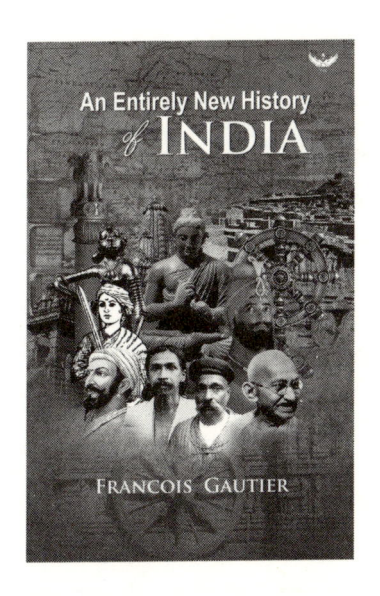

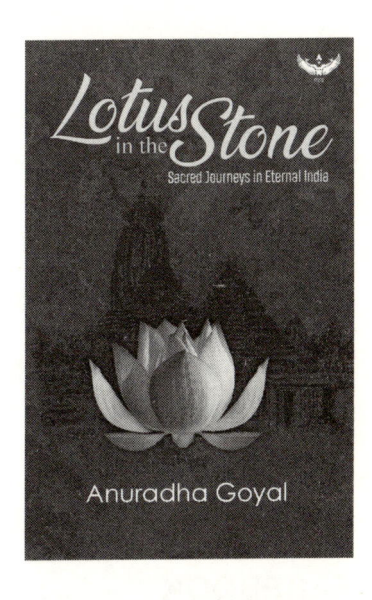

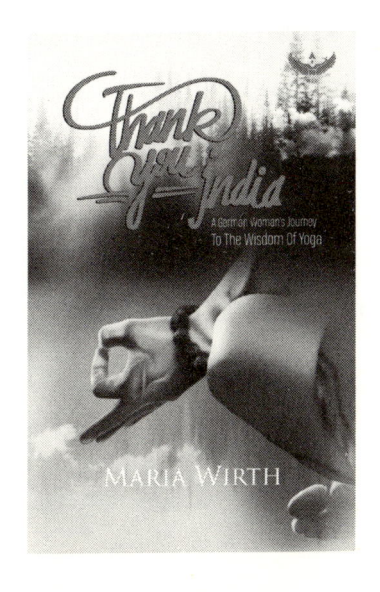

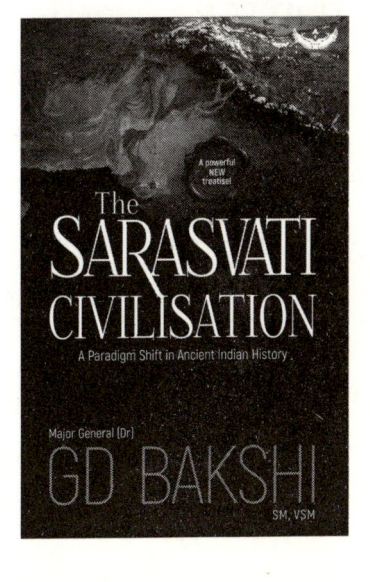

An Entirely New History of INDIA
Francois Gautier

Lotus in the Stone
Sacred Journeys in Eternal India
Anuradha Goyal

Thank You India
A German Woman's Journey To The Wisdom Of Yoga
Maria Wirth

The SARASVATI CIVILISATION
A Paradigm Shift in Ancient Indian History
Major General (Dr) **GD BAKSHI**
SM, VSM

गरुड

Register:

Please register your book purchase at **grpr.in/register** to stay in touch and get informed about future books!

To order:
www.garudabooks.com

Follow us:

WEBSITE : www.garudabooks.com
FACEBOOK : www.facebook.com/garudaprakashan/
TWITTER : @garudaprakashan
INSTAGRAM: @garudabooks
YOUTUBE : /garudabooks

Contact:

EMAIL : contact@garudabooks.com

International queries:

EMAIL : international@garudabooks.com